D1613936

Periodontal Regeneration Enhanced

Clinical Applications of Enamel Matrix Proteins

Periodontal Regeneration Enhanced

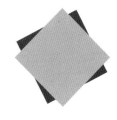

Clinical Applications of Enamel Matrix Proteins

Thomas G. Wilson, Jr, DDS
Private Practice, Periodontics and Dental Implants
Dallas, Texas

Quintessence Publishing Co, Inc
Chicago, Berlin, London, Tokyo, Paris, Barcelona, São Paulo,
Moscow, Prague, and Warsaw

Library of Congress Cataloging-in-Publication Data

Wilson, Thomas G.
    Periodontal regeneration enhanced : clinical applications of enamel
  matrix proteins / Thomas G. Wilson, Jr.
       p.   cm.
    Includes bibliographical references.
    ISBN 0-86715-352-0
    1. Periodontium—Regeneration.   2. Dental enamel—Physiology.
  I. Title.
    [DNLM: 1. Periodontal Diseases—therapy.   2. Dental Enamel
Proteins—therapeutic use.   3. Guided Tissue Regeneration—methods.
  WU 240 W753p 1999]
  RK361.W55 1999
  617.6'32—dc21
  DNLM/DLC
  for Library of Congress   98-47492
                                        CIP

quintessence
books

© 1999 Quintessence Publishing Co, Inc

Quintessence Publishing Co, Inc
551 Kimberly Drive
Carol Stream, Illinois 60188

Editor: Cheryl Anderson-Wiedenbeck
Production: Timothy M. Robbins
Design: Michael Shanahan

Printed in China

Contents

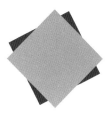

To my family, Penny, Trey, and John, and to my mother.
How do you guys put up with all this stuff?

Dental science is an ever-changing field.
It is important for the reader to keep abreast of new material
as it is published and to update the material presented in this text.

Preface

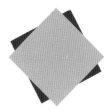

Reducing pathologically deepened probing depths is a laudable goal. When and how to best approach these bacterial sumps is the quandary. While closed procedures are effective in controlling some, in many cases surgery is warranted.

Over the last few years the emphasis of surgical procedures has shifted more and more toward regeneration with the idea that this would increase the longevity of the dentition. While the dental profession has made strides toward improving these surgical techniques and procedures, predictability in achieving new attachment is often lacking.

This book is about the use of enamel matrix proteins, which represent the next step toward more predictable regeneration. These proteins have regularly produced positive soft and hard tissue reactions not seen by the author when using other regenerative approaches and, in the author's opinion, warrant more widespread attention from clinicians.

Acknowledgments

The author would like to thank Professor Lars Hammerström for his expertise; Drs Lars Heijl, Stina Gestrelius, and Otis Bouwsma for their contributions in writing and editing; Dr Martha Somerman for her advice and counsel; Terry Cockerham for his wonderful drawings; Trey Wilson for his help in composing the material; and, of course, Georgia Wright for her organizational and typing skills.

Basic Science of Enamel Matrix Proteins

The placement of enamel matrix proteins on a properly prepared tooth surface during surgery can result in significant regeneration of lost periodontal tissues. Enamel matrix proteins play an important role in tooth development and have been found to have virtually the same molecular structure in all mammalian species studied thus far. The proteins are harvested from around developing teeth in carefully selected young pigs and, following special processing procedures, are packaged for use in dentistry under the trade name Emdogain (Biora). Most of the initial work with this material has been aimed at regenerating periodontal attachment apparatus lost due to periodontitis (Figs 1-1 to 1-6), but other applications are being explored.

Regeneration Versus Repair

By definition, regeneration is the reproduction or reconstitution of a lost or injured part.[1] For the purposes of this text, *regeneration* is the formation of new cementum, periodontal ligament, and alveolar bone following periodontal surgery after

pathologic exposure of the root surface has occurred secondary to inflammatory periodontal diseases (Figs 1-7a to 1-7d). Regeneration is important because it is widely assumed that the tissues generated during this process are more resistant to breakdown than tissues obtained where healing occurs by repair.

Repair can be defined as the healing of a wound by tissue that does not fully restore the previous architecture or function (Figs 1-8a to 1-8c). Specifically, repair is the form of healing found most often following periodontal procedures not specifically aimed at producing regeneration. Most (approximately 90% of) healing along the root seen following flap surgery is by repair. This surgical approach usually results in a long junctional epithelium or, at best, a combination of a long junctional epithelium and a long connective tissue attachment.

In the author's experience and that of others,[2] tissues that have healed by repair are more subject to continued attachment loss than those generated by surgical procedures designed to produce regeneration. In addition, healing by repair does not result in restoration of the original form (new cementum, periodontal ligament, and alveolar bone), nor is original function of the periodontal attachment apparatus restored.

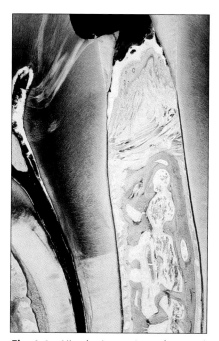

Fig 1-1a Histologic section of normal human periodontium. Note the relationship of the bone, periodontal ligament, and cementum. (Original magnification ×3.2.) (Photo courtesy Dr Robert Schenk. From material provided by Dr Gisbert Krekeler.)

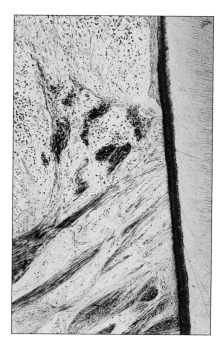

Fig 1-1b Closer view of the section seen in Fig 1-1a. There are minimal numbers of inflammatory cells and there is no proliferation of the junctional epithelium. (Original magnification ×25.) (Photo courtesy Dr Robert Schenk. From material provided by Dr Gisbert Krekeler.)

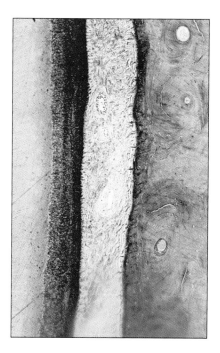

Fig 1-2 Section of normal human attachment apparatus made up of acellular cementum, periodontal ligament, and alveolar bone seen at ×25 magnification. (Photo courtesy Dr Robert Schenk. From material provided by Dr Gisbert Krekeler.)

Fig 1-3a Buccolingual cross section of a tooth and normal periodontium.

Fig 1-3b Magnified view of the normal tooth seen in Fig 1-3a. E = enamel, S = gingival sulcus, JE = junctional epithelium, D = dentin, C = cementum, AB = alveolar bone, PDL = periodontal ligament.

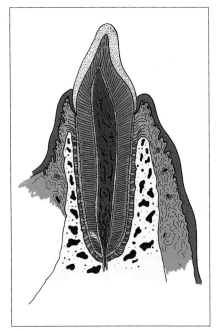

Fig 1-3a

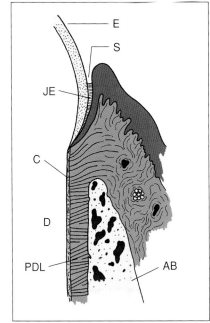

Fig 1-3b

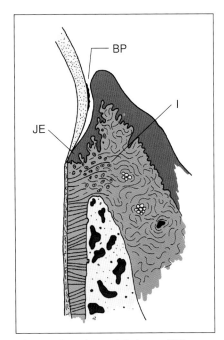

Fig 1-4 Once bacterial plaque (BP) accumulates in the gingival sulcus, gingivitis results. This is characterized by inflammatory cells (I) in the area just adjacent to the junctional epithelium (JE).

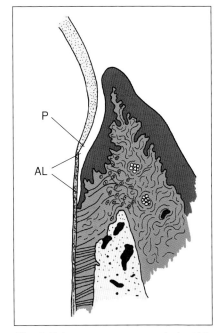

Fig 1-5 In some cases periodontitis follows gingivitis. The hallmarks of periodontitis are attachment loss (AL), meaning loss of periodontal ligament and alveolar bone, and pocket (P) formation.

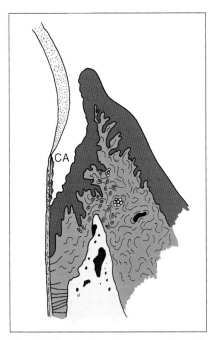

Fig 1-6 Root alterations seen in periodontitis, including accumulations of bacterial plaque and calculus (CA). Such alterations result in a hypermineralized root surface that masks the connective tissue fibers needed to reattach the fibers of the PDL during regeneration.

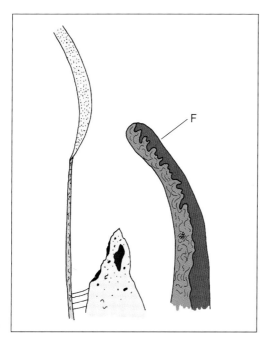

Fig 1-7a To most predictably regenerate lost periodontal attachment (new cementum, periodontal ligament, and bone), a gingival flap (F) is raised and the root surface is prepared.

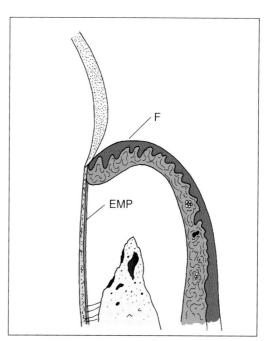

Fig 1-7b The root surface is coated with enamel matrix proteins (EMP) and the flap (F) is sutured in place. Space maintenance is usually not needed. (Compare to Fig 2-2c.)

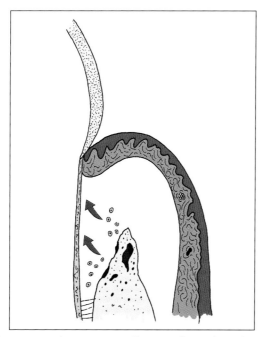

Fig 1-7c For regeneration to occur, cells must migrate from the PDL and the area of the alveolar bone to cover the previously diseased root surface.

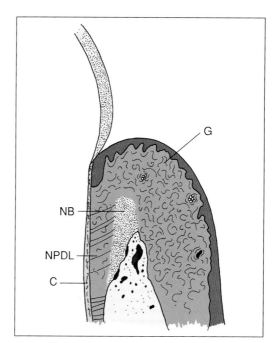

Fig 1-7d The desired endpoint of this process is new bone (NB), new periodontal ligament (NPDL), and new cementum (C), along with normal architecture and attachment of the gingival tissues (G).

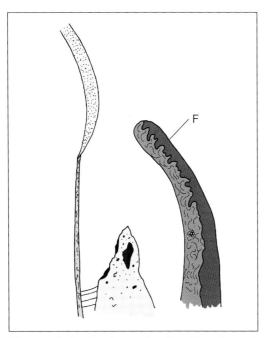

Fig 1-8a In healing by repair, a flap (F) is elevated and the root surface prepared.

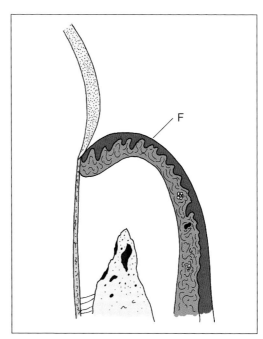

Fig 1-8b The flap (F) is then replaced and sutured. No additional attempt is made to achieve regeneration.

Fig 1-8c Healing by repair usually results in a long junctional epithelial attachment (LJE) and some new bone (NB). This process often produces a small amount of new attachment (NA).

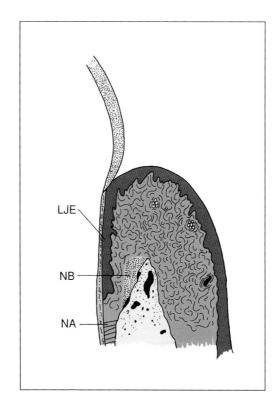

Importance of Cementum

Of the three tissues resulting from regeneration, the formation of cementum plays an early and critical role. Cementum is essential for the maintenance of the periodontal attachment apparatus because it traps the connective tissue fibers that attach the tooth to bone.

There are different types of cementum based on the presence or absence of cells and the origin and direction of trapped fibers.[3] The middle two thirds of the root surface in humans is normally covered by a thin layer of acellular cementum (including extrinsic fiber cementum; see Fig 1-2a), while the remainder of the root is covered by cellular cementum. Cellular mixed stratified cementum, which is composed of extrinsic and intrinsic fibers and irregularly distributed cells, is usually found in the apical one third of the root. Acellular, afibrillar cementum contains neither cells nor fibers and is part of the acellular extrinsic fiber cementum.[4] Other types of cementum are also found. Cellular intrinsic cementum contains cells and collagenous fibers, but the fibers do not extend into the periodontal ligament. This tissue is mainly associated with repair following root resorption.

This text focuses on acellular extrinsic fiber cementum, because this tissue is primarily responsible for the connection of tooth to alveolar bone by means of the periodontal ligament before loss of periodontal attachment occurs. Regeneration of this type of cementum is one of the goals of therapy because this tissue appears to provide the most tenacious anchor of periodontal ligament fibers to the tooth.[5]

Development of Attachment Apparatus

Cementum is first laid down during tooth development. The stimulus for this development comes from the remnants of the epithelial root sheath (ERS), also called Hertwig's epithelial root sheath. The ERS induces mesenchymal cells of the dental papilla to form predentin (Figs 1-9a to 1-9c). When the mesenchymal cells of the dental follicle are exposed to products of the ERS, these cells appear to produce enamel matrix proteins that stimulate undifferentiated mesenchymal cells to form cementoblasts. Cementoblasts then lay down cementum on the predentin of the developing root (Figs 1-9d and 1-9e).[6] (For a review, see Bosshardt and Schroeder.[7])

The idea that the phenomenon of cementoblast differentiation is stimulated by what are now termed enamel matrix proteins related to the ERS was first proposed by Slavkin in 1976[8] and Schonfeld and Slavkin in 1977[9] and was confirmed by subsequent studies.[10-12] The proteins of the enamel matrix can be divided into two major groups: the amelogenins and the enamelins.

The amelogenins make up 90% of these proteins, with the remaining 10% containing proline-rich enamelin, tuftelin, tuft protein, serum proteins, and at least one salivary protein.[4] It is important to know that amelogenins of similar molecular structure have been found in many different mammalian species,[13] including humans, which allows compatibility between species.

Deposition of enamel matrix proteins on the root surface sets in motion a series of events that leads to generation of the periodontal attachment apparatus. This consists of connective tissue fibers (later called Sharpey's fibers) that become trapped along with alveolar bone and cementum. This process takes many months to completely surround the developing tooth (Fig 1-9f).[14-19]

The enamel matrix proteins and their applications in dentistry are the subject of this text.

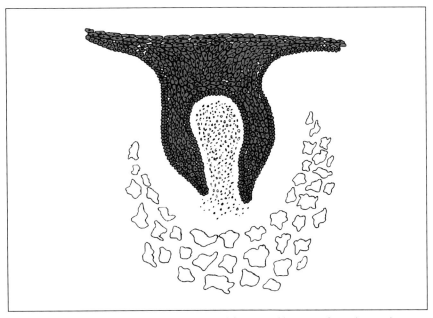

Fig 1-9a The cells of the oral epithelium proliferate and begin to form the tooth.

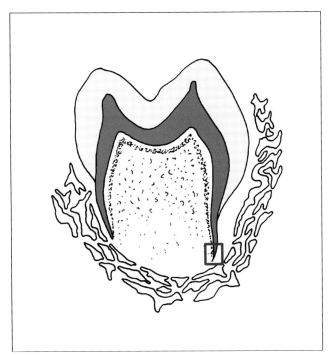

Fig 1-9b Following formation of the crown of the tooth, the epithelial root sheath (ERS) continues to proliferate apically.

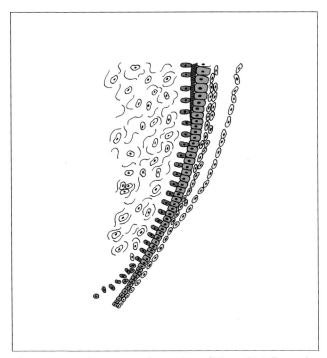

Fig 1-9c An enlargement of a section of Fig 1-9b. Cells on the tooth side of the ERS stimulate mesenchymal cells to form predentin. Other cells of the ERS stimulate mesenchymal cells to form cementoblasts.

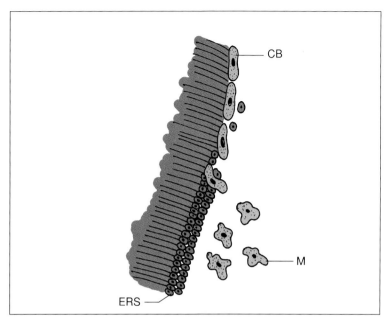

Fig 1-9d An enlargement of the apical portion of the ERS. M = mesenchymal cells, ERS = epithelial root sheath, CB = cementoblasts.

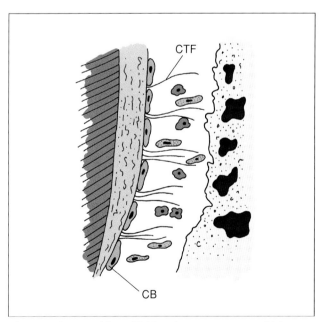

Fig 1-9e Cementoblasts (CB) lay down cementum, which traps connective tissue fibers (CTF).

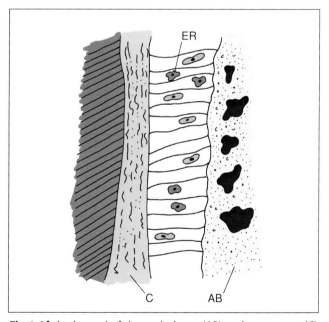

Fig 1-9f At the end of the cycle, bone (AB) and cementum (C) are linked by the periodontal ligament. The remnants of the ERS are often referred to as the epithelial rest of Malassez (ER).

References

1. American Academy of Periodontology. Glossary of Periodontal Terms, ed 3. Chicago: American Academy of Periodontology, 1992:46.

2. Waerhaug J. In discussion following Elleguard B: New Attachment as an Objective of Surgery. In: Shanley DB (ed). Efficacy of Treatment in Periodontics. Chicago: Quintessence, 1980:145.

3. Listgarten MA, Kamin A. The development of a cementum layer over the enamel surface of rabbit molars. A light and electron microscopic study. Arch Oral Biol 1969;14:961.

4. Hammarström L. Enamel matrix, cementum development and regeneration. J Clin Periodontol 1997;24: 658.

5. Schröeder H. Biological problems of regenerative cementogenesis: Synthesis and attachment of collagenous matrices on growing and established root surface. Int Rev Cytol 1992;142:1.

6. Paynter KJ, Pudy G. A study of the structure, chemical nature and development of cementum in the rat. Anat Rec 1958;131:233.

7. Bosshardt DD, Schröeder HE. Cementogenesis reviewed. A comparison between human premolars and rodent molars. Anat Rec 1996;245:267.

8. Slavkin HC. Towards a cellular and molecular understanding of periodontics: Cementogenesis revisited. J Periodontol 1976;47:249.

9. Schonfeld SE, Slavkin HC. Demonstration of enamel matrix proteins on root-analogue surfaces of rabbit permanent incisor teeth. Calcif Tissue Res 1977;24:223.

10. Lindskog S. Formation of intermediate cementum (I). Early mineralization of aprismatic enamel and intermediate cementum in monkey. J Craniofac Genet Dev Biol 1982;2:147.

11. Lindskog S. Formation of intermediate cementum (II). A scanning electron microscopic study of the epithelial root sheath of Hertwig in monkey. J Craniofac Genet Dev Biol 1982;2:161.

12. Lindskog S, Hammarström L. Formation of intermediate cementum III: 3H-tryptophane and 3H-proline uptake into the epithelial root sheath of Hertwig in vitro. J Craniofac Genet Dev Biol 1982;2:172.

13. Brookes SJ, Robinson C, Kirkham J, Bonass WA. Biochemistry and molecular biology of amelogenin proteins of developing dental enamel. Arch Oral Biol 1995;40:1.

14. Hammarström L. The role of enamel matrix proteins in the development of cementum and periodontal tissues. In: 1997 Dental Enamel. Ciba Foundation Symposium 205. 1997;246.

15. MacNeil RL, Berry J, D'Errico J, Strayhorn C, Somerman M. Localization and expression of osteopontin in mineralized and non-mineralized tissues of the periodontium. Ann N Y Acad Sci 1995;760:166.

16. Pitaru S, McCulloch CAG, Narayanan SA. Cellular origins and differentiation control mechanisms during periodontal development and wound healing. J Periodontal Res 1994;29:81.

17. McCulloch CAG. Basic considerations in periodontal wound healing to achieve regeneration. Periodontology 2000 1993;1:16.

18. Aukhil I, Nishimura K, Fernyhough W. Experimental regeneration of the periodontium. Crit Rev Oral Biol Med 1990;1:101.

19. Nanci A, McKee MD, Smith CE (eds). The biology of dental tissues. Anat Rec 1996(special issue);245.

Evolution of Methods to Achieve Regeneration

Regeneration of periodontal attachment apparatus lost to disease or trauma is a worthy goal for at least three reasons. The first is that with regeneration comes pocket depth reduction and the concomitant reduction of the aggressive pathogens typically found in deep pockets. The second is the increased possibility that the patient, with good personal oral hygiene, will be able to more predictably disrupt the organization of subgingival bacterial plaque, thus preventing its maturity and subsequent increased pathogenicity. The third reason is that shallow pockets are easier for the dental professional to maintain.

Because regeneration is by definition a rebirth of the periodontium, it can add longevity to the dentition; however, achieving this goal is not simple. Attempts to make it a predictable clinical reality have taken numerous forms, and approaches continue to evolve. As detailed in this chapter, enamel matrix proteins are an important step in this progress.

Initial Approaches to Obtaining Regeneration

Dentistry currently strives for regeneration, not repair. This trend started when traditional surgical and nonsurgical approaches were found to produce minimal amounts of new periodontal attachment apparatus.[1–3] Specifically, closed subgingival scaling and root planing in humans has been shown to produce little regeneration.[4] The same was true for surgery using a replaced flap.[5] (See chapter 1 for details on this process.)

It was subsequently suggested that the addition of various graft materials might increase the amount of new bone, periodontal ligament (PDL), and cementum generated. Although this approach often produced good clinical results,[6] there was little true regeneration when studied histologically. In fact, it was demonstrated in both humans and animals that a downgrowth of the junctional epithelium (ie, formation of a long junctional epithelium) close to the base of the original defect occurs when bone grafts alone are used (Fig 2-1).[7,8]

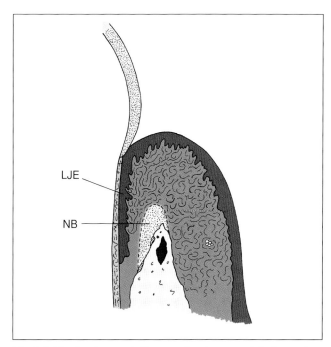

Fig 2-1 Healing by repair. Bone grafts alone result in formation of new bone (NB), but a long junctional epithelium (LJE) is often found between the bone and the tooth surface.

Obtaining good clinical results is an important objective, and many dentitions were no doubt saved with procedures that produced minimal amounts of true regeneration. Even so, the goal of finding a predictable regenerative procedure remained elusive. Clinically, it is impossible to know whether or not regeneration has occurred because histology is the only reliable method for determining the nature of the new tissues formed following therapy.

A reasonable method for determining true regeneration in histologic studies is the use of a notch placed in the tooth at the apical extent of the calculus. New bone, PDL, and cementum must be produced coronal to this notch to signify that a regenerative event took place.[9] When this method proved that traditional surgical and nonsurgical methods as well as bone grafting were unreliable for producing significant amounts of regeneration,

other directions were explored. The next advance toward achieving more predictable regeneration was provided by guided tissue regeneration.

Guided Tissue Regeneration

Guided tissue regeneration (GTR) depends on the exclusion of the gingival tissues from the root surface during the first few months following surgery (Figs 2-2a to 2-2e). Barrier membranes are used to block the cells of the gingival tissues and create an area under the membranes for regeneration to occur.[10] This approach allows cell proliferation in the area of the periodontal ligament and around the alveolar bone. Cells are expected to migrate up the tooth root and regenerate the desired tissues.[10–12]

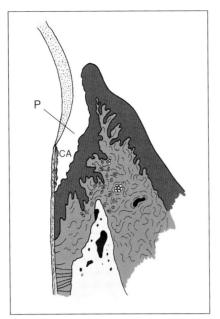

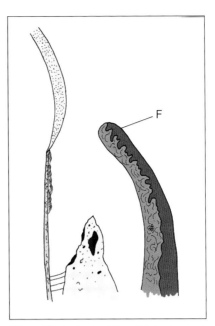

Fig 2-2a Alterations seen as a result of periodontitis. Pocket formation (P) is evident, as are calculus (CA) and other bacterial products on the root surface.

Fig 2-2b A gingival flap (F) is elevated and the root prepared as in other regenerative procedures.

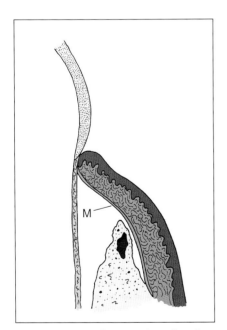

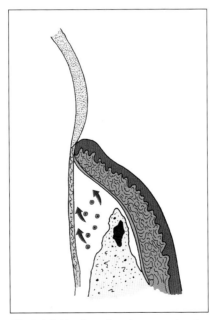

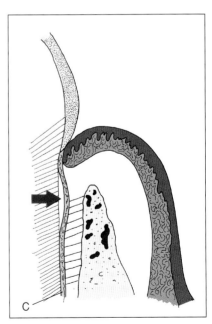

Fig 2-2c A membrane (M) is placed to exclude the gingival tissue during healing and to create space for a blood clot to form.

Fig 2-2d Ideally, cells migrate under the membrane and create new attachment (acellular cementum, PDL, and bone).

Fig 2-2e Even if the procedure is successful, the cementum (C) produced is often cellular and may tear away when processed histologically *(arrow)*.

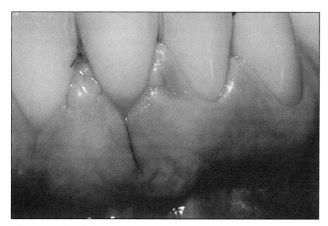

Fig 2-3a Guided tissue regeneration using an e-PTFE membrane. This patient presented with deep pockets around a mandibular central incisor that had received endodontic therapy.

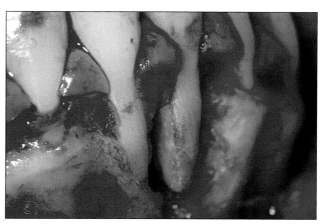

Fig 2-3b The flap was reflected and the area debrided.

The procedure begins with elevation of a flap, followed by debridement of the root surface. The membrane is then placed and covered with the flap to exclude the gingival tissues. Most of the early work with this technique used nonabsorbable barrier membranes, notably expanded polytetraethylfluorethylene (e-PTFE)[13] (Figs 2-3a to 2-3f). It is important to note that the use of enamel matrix proteins, in contradistinction to achieving regeneration with GTR in smaller defects, does *not* require space maintenance.

Positive clinical results using GTR are difficult to achieve because success depends on a complex series of steps to prepare the root surface[14] and then to place and secure the membrane.[10] After the membrane has been placed, care must also be taken to avoid bacterial contamination of the membrane until it is scheduled for removal.

On a cellular level, success also depends on a complex series of events involving the proliferation of the targeted cell populations. It has been suggested that seven steps are needed to successfully complete the process of regeneration on the cellular level[15]:

1. The infected tissues must be eliminated and the healing site kept free of pathogens.
2. Populations of progenitor cells must be adjacent to the wound site.
3. The progenitor cells must differentiate and then proliferate.
4. These new cells must migrate to appropriate sites on the tooth surface.
5. Once migrated, the new cells must establish cell populations that will be responsible for long-term tissue maintenance of the attachment apparatus.
6. The new cells must organize in a manner that will result in formation of a new attachment apparatus.
7. The new cells must then establish homeostasis.

The use of nonabsorbable membranes poses problems for the clinician. One problem is these membranes must be removed at a second surgery. This is often an elaborate and time-consuming step, and requires additional trauma for the patient. Another problem is the membranes frequently become exposed, in spite of the clinician's best

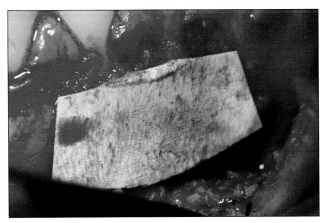

Fig 2-3c Freeze-dried human bone was placed in the defect and covered with an e-PTFE membrane.

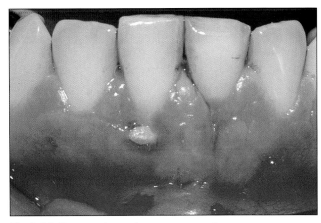

Fig 2-3d The membrane became exposed.

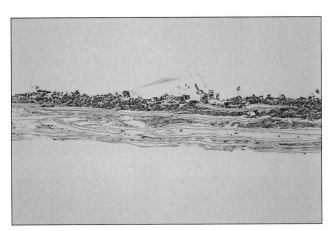

Fig 2-3e Bacterial infiltration of the membrane could be seen following its surgical removal.

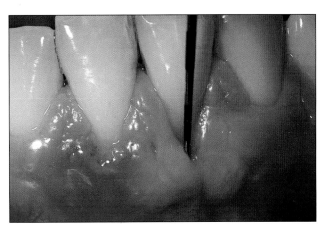

Fig 2-3f The area 5 years following surgery. The bony defect is gone and the probing depths are within normal limits.

attempts to avoid this. Premature exposure (before 3 months) means that bacteria may infiltrate the membrane.[16] Exposure and premature removal of membranes usually leads to less desirable clinical and histologic results.[17]

The desire to leave the surgical site undisturbed by a second surgery led to the development of multiple types of absorbable barriers, including collagen, cargile membranes, polylactic acid, oxidized cellulose, Vicryl, and others.[18] Although clinical success has been reported with all of these materials, there is still a great deal that is not known about some of the mechanisms of absorption, and histologic confirmation of their ability to routinely produce significant amounts of regeneration and long-term clinical success is scarce.[19] Bacterial contamination of these membranes also has been reported.[20]

Although the initial clinical results using GTR are often good, increasing breakdown of the sites over time has been reported.[21–23] Some of the results seem to depend on patient compliance. Not surprisingly, the better the compliance with suggested plaque control procedures and maintenance visits, the more stable the results of the GTR.[22,23] However, other factors also may contribute to the breakdown. Instead of producing acellular cementum, which would constitute "true" regeneration, cellular cementum is often found as a product of GTR. During processing for histologic evaluation, tears are often noted between the cellular cementum and the fibers of the periodontal ligament. This may indicate that the attachment thus formed is not as strong as that seen following true regeneration.[24,25]

Attempts have been made to increase the success of clinical outcomes for GTR by combining membranes with various graft materials. The use of freeze-dried bone plus e-PTFE membranes gave superior clinical furcation closure (72%) in Class II furcations compared to that found with e-PTFE membranes alone (31%).[26] In another study, only 13% of the Class II furcations studied closed when treated with freeze-dried bone and membranes,[27] whereas others found no difference in results in closing furcations when bone grafts plus membranes were compared to membranes alone.[28] No additional benefit was found in using graft materials with absorbable membranes.[29,30]

Only a limited number of published reports on human histology have evaluated membranes and graft materials. In one study, porous hydroxyapatite was used along with an e-PTFE membrane; no evidence was found of new attachment coronal to the notch made at the apical extent of calculus at the time of surgery.[31] Stahl and coworkers found new attachment in 6 out of 9 human defects,[32] in 3 out of 4 human suprabony sites,[33] and in 2 out of 4 human vertical lesion sites.[34]

It can generally be said that guided tissue regeneration in its present form has allowed the prolonged retention of treated teeth, but it has failed to give the profession a predictable method for regeneration of lost periodontal attachment apparatus. This is because the classic use of this approach, while often resulting in cellular cementum and new connective tissue attachment, usually lacks sufficient amounts of either acellular cementum or new alveolar bone for significant regeneration or lacks proper orientation of the reproduced elements.[35–40] The amount of new cementum produced ranged from 100% in all defects where the teeth were completely covered by soft tissue[40] to virtually 0%[38] where teeth were not covered but had coronally positioned flaps. Other variations included a 2% value reported by Haney et al and 0% to 75% new cementum reported by Sigurdsson et al.[35]

Growth Factors

The future holds even more possibilities for materials that may enhance the clinician's ability to produce regeneration. One such approach may be the use of growth factors. Growth factors are proteins found in various tissues that play a major role in wound healing. In general, these molecules seem to have an important role in such events as migration, attachment, and proliferation of nearly all cell types.[41] Recently, various combinations of these materials have been used for regeneration. Although some of the results look very promising, thus far use of growth factors in periodontal therapy has largely been limited to in vitro and animal studies,[42] and several important questions need to be resolved before these materials are used routinely in the clinic.[43]

The uncertainty of the clinical outcomes for the procedures already discussed in this chapter has led many clinicians to seek other, more predictable methods to obtain regeneration than are currently available. This has set the stage for the use of enamel matrix proteins.

Enamel Matrix Proteins

Hammarström et al[44] used a monkey model in which a flap was raised on the facial aspect of the mandibular teeth and all the bone, periodontal ligament, and cementum were removed. After the teeth were treated with acid to remove the smear layer, various preparations of enamel matrix proteins were placed with or without carrier vehicles. Eight weeks following surgery, the teeth were removed in block sections.

The best results were obtained in the sites where a combination of propylene glycol alginate (PGA) was used as a vehicle along with enamel matrix proteins (the proteins found in Emdogain). At these test sites there was, on average, 70% new cementum and 65% bone gain (Figs 2-4a and 2-4b). At the control sites, where only carrier PGA had been used, there was 10% new cementum and 10% bone gain.

Additional histologic evidence, this time human, was provided by Heijl.[45] Following the surgical removal of the periodontal attachment apparatus on the facial aspect of a mandibular human incisor and placement of Emdogain, healing was allowed to proceed for 4 months. The tooth was then removed for orthodontic purposes. The block section revealed 74% new cementum and 65% bone gain on the previously denuded root surface (Figs 2-5a and 2-5b).

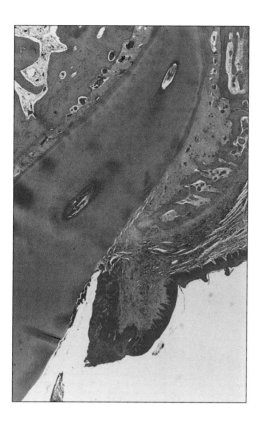

Fig 2-4a A monkey maxillary premolar 8 weeks after surgery which removed the alveolar bone, periodontal ligament, and cementum. A significant portion of the attachment apparatus has regenerated following placement of enamel matrix proteins. (From Hammarström L, et al.[44] Reproduced with permission from Munksgaard International Publishers.)

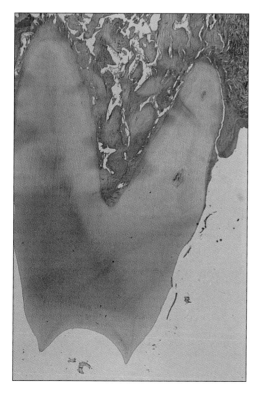

Fig 2-4b A premolar treated in a manner similar to that in Fig 2-4a, but without the use of enamel matrix proteins. Minimal new attachment has occurred. (From Hammarström L, et al.[44] Reproduced with permission from Munksgaard International Publishers.)

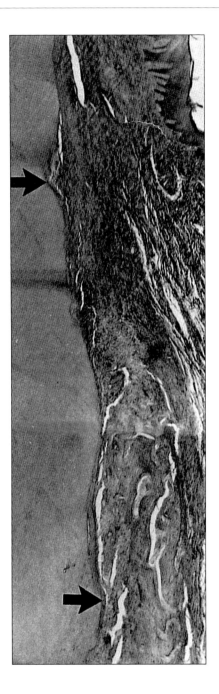

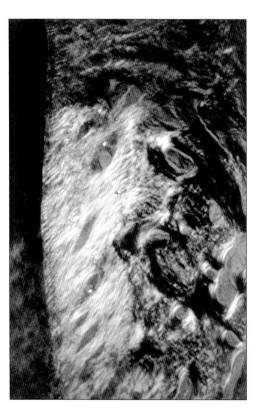

Fig 2-5a *(Left)* Human histologic section taken after the attachment apparatus had been surgically removed 4 months previously. (From Heijl L.[45] Reproduced with permission from Munksgaard International Publishers.)

Fig 2-5b *(Below)* The new acellular cementum, periodontal ligament, and alveolar bone found following placement of enamel matrix proteins. The case is the same as in Fig 2-5a. (From Heijl L.[45] Reproduced with permission from Munksgaard International Publishers.)

Heijl et al[46] used 34 paired interproximal test and control sites that were primarily one- or two-wall bony defects. In this three-year study, attachment levels, radiographic bone levels, and probing depths were measured. A split-mouth design was used with randomly selected test and control sites. All clinical measurements were made by blinded examiners. There were three study centers with a total of 35 patients. A placebo consisting of the carrier vehicle (PGA) was placed on the control side and the test enamel matrix protein material on the other. Only interproximal sites with probe depths of 6 mm or greater and radiographic bony lesions of 4 × 2 mm or greater were studied.

The results showed that on the test sites the pocket depths were reduced 3.1 mm, while on the control sites they were reduced 2.3 mm. The clinical attachment in the test sites gained 2.2 mm compared to 1.7 mm in the control sites. On radiographs, there was a 2.6-mm bone gain at the test sites whereas the control sites showed a small net loss of bone.

One study compared GTR with the use of enamel matrix proteins in the treatment of artificially created Class III furcations in dogs.[47] Resolut Regenerative Material (WL Gore) was the control and Emdogain, using 37% phosphoric acid for 15 seconds, was the test. Similar amounts of mineralized bone marrow and periodontal ligament tissue were formed in both groups. New acellular cementum was found only in the apical portion of the test defects.

It can be said that enamel matrix proteins (Emdogain) have produced positive clinical and histologic results. They have routinely produced 60% to 70% new bone, periodontal ligament, and acellular cementum in histologic studies. The studies discussed in this section are the basis for far-ranging laboratory and clinical trials now being conducted on the material for a variety of clinical applications. If the available data is confirmed, enamel matrix proteins will provide an excellent alternative to current methods and will allow the clinician to more predictably achieve true periodontal regeneration. In addition, the utility of the proteins may be expanded for other types of periodontal therapy.

References

1. Bowers G, Chadroff B, Carnevale R, et al. Histologic evaluation of new attachment apparatus formation in humans, Part I. J Periodontol 1989;60(12):664.

2. Bowers G, Chadroff B, Carnevale R, et al. Histologic evaluation of new attachment apparatus formation in humans, Part III. J Periodontol 1989;60(12):683.

3. Fowler C, Garrett S, Crigger M, Egelberg J. Histological probe position in treated and untreated human periodontal tissues. J Clin Periodontol 1982;9(5):373.

4. Dragoo M. Closed curettage. In: Dragoo M (ed). Regeneration of the Periodontal Attachment in Humans. Philadelphia: Lea and Febinger, 1981:35.

5. Steiner SS, Crigger M, Egelberg J. Connective tissue regeneration to periodontally diseased teeth. II. Histologic observation of cases following replaced flap surgery. J Periodontal Res 1981;16:109.

6. Schallhorn RG. Long-term evaluation of osseous grafts in periodontal therapy. Int Dent J 1980;30:101.

7. Cator JG, Zander HA. Osseous repair of an infrabony pocket without new attachment of connective tissue. J Clin Periodontol 1976;3:54.

8. Listgarten MA, Rosenberg MM. Histological study of repair following new attachment procedures in human periodontal lesions. J Periodontol 1979;50(7):333.

9. Cole RT, Crigger M, Bogle G, Egelberg J, Selvig KA. Connective tissue regeneration to periodontally diseased teeth. J Periodontal Res 1980;15:1.

10. Nyman S, Gottlow J, Karring T, Lindhe J. The regenerative potential of the periodontal ligament. An experimental study in the monkey. J Clin Periodontol 1982;9(3):257.

11. Melcher AH, McCulloch CAG, Cheong T, Nemeth E, Shiga A. Cells from bone synthesize cementum-like and bone-like tissue in vitro and may migrate into periodontal ligament in vivo. J Periodontal Res 1987;22:246.

12. Melcher AH. On the repair potential of periodontal tissues. J Periodontol 1976;47:256.

13. Gottlow J, Nyman S, Lindhe J, Karring T, Wennstrom J. New attachment formation in the human periodontium by guided tissue regeneration. Case reports. J Clin Periodontol 1986;13(6):604.

14. Polson AM, Caton J. Factors influencing periodontal repair and regeneration. J Periodontol 1982;53:617.

15. McCulloch CAG. Basic considerations in periodontal wound healing to achieve regeneration. Periodontology 2000 1993;1:16.

16. Simion M, Trisi P, Maglione M, Piattelli A. Bacterial penetration in vitro through GTAM membranes with and without topical chlorhexidine application. J Clin Periodontol 1995;22:321.

17. Selvig KA, Kersten B, Chamberlain ADH, Wikesjö UME, Nilveus RE. Regenerative surgery of intrabony periodontal defects using ePTFE membranes. J Periodontol 1992;63:974.

18. Greenstein G, Caton JG. Biodegradable barriers and guided tissue regeneration. Periodontology 2000 1993;1:36.

19. Magnusson I, Stenberg WV, Batich C, Egelberg J. Connective tissue repair in circumferential periodontal defects in dogs following use of a biodegradable membrane. J Clin Periodontol 1990;17:243.

20. Wang HL, Kuo Y, Burgett F, Shyr Y, Sued S. Adherence of microorganisms to guided tissue regeneration membranes. An in vitro study. J Periodontol 1994;65:211.

21. Gottlow J, Nyman S, Karring T. Maintenance of new attachment gained through guided tissue regeneration. J Clin Periodontol 1992;19:315.

22. Cortellini P, Pini-Prato G, Tonetti M. Periodontal regeneration of human infrabony defect (V). Effect of oral hygiene on long-term stability. J Clin Periodontol 1994;21:606.

23. Weigel C, Bragger U, Hammerle CHF, Mombelli A, Lang NP. Maintenance of new attachment 1 and 4 years following guided tissue regeneration (GTR). J Clin Periodontol 1995;22(9):661.

24. Schroeder H. Biological problems of regenerative cementogenesis: Synthesis and attachment of collagenous matrices on growing and established root surface. Int Rev Cytol 1992;142:1.

25. de Araujo F, Berglundh T, Lindhe J. The periodontal tissues in healed degree III furcation defects. An experimental study in dogs. J Clin Periodontol 1996;23:532.

26. Schallhorn RG, McClain PK. Long-term assessment of combined osseous composite grafting, root conditioning, and guided tissue regeneration. Int J Periodontics Restorative Dent 1993;13:9.

27. Anderegg C, Martin S, Gray J, Mellonig J, Gher M. Clinical evaluation of the use of decalcified freeze-dried bone allograft with guided tissue regeneration in the treatment of molar furcation invasions. J Periodontol 1991;62:264.

28. Walleye SC, Gellin RG, Miller MC, Mishkin DJ. Guided tissue regeneration with and without decalcified freeze-dried bone in mandibular class II furcation invasions. J Periodontol 1994;65:244.

29. Chen CC, Wang HL, Smith F, Glickman GN, Shyr Y, O'Neal RB. Evaluation of a collagen membrane with and without bone grafts in treating periodontal intrabony defects. J Periodontol 1995;66:838.

30. Blumenthal NM, Steinberg J. The use of collagen membrane barriers in conjunction with combined demineralized bone-collagen gel implants in human intrabony defects. J Periodontol 1990;61:319.

31. Stahl SS, Froum S. Human intrabony lesion responses to debridement, porous hydroxyapatite implants and Teflon barrier membranes. J Clin Periodontol 1991; 18:605.

32. Stahl SS, Froum SJ, Tarnow D. Human histologic responses to guided tissue regeneration techniques in intrabony lesions. J Clin Periodontol 1990;17:191.

33. Stahl SS, Froum S. Healing of suprabony lesions treated with guided tissue regeneration and coronally anchored flaps. Case reports. J Clin Periodontol 1991;18:69.

34. Stahl SS, Froum S. Histologic healing responses in human vertical lesions following the use of osseous allografts and barrier membranes. J Clin Periodontol 1991;18:149.

35. Sigurdsson TJ, Hardwick R, Bogle GC, Wikesjö UME. Periodontal repair in dogs: Space provision by reinforced ePTFE membranes enhance bone and cementum regeneration in large supraalveolar defects. J Periodontol 1994;65:350.

36. Wikesjö UM, Sigurdsson TJ, Lee MB, Tatkis DN, Selvig KA. Dynamics of wound healing in periodontal regenerative therapy. J Calif Dent Assoc 1995;23(12):30.

37. Haney JM, Nilveus RE, McMillan PJ, Wikesjö UME. Periodontal repair in dogs: Expanded polytetrafluorethylene barrier membranes support wound stabilization and enhance bone regeneration. J Periodontol 1993;64:883.

38. Wikesjö UME, Nilveus R. Periodontal repair in dogs: Healing patterns in large circumferential periodontal defects. J Clin Periodontol 1991;18:49.

39. Caton JG, DeFuria EL, Polson AM, Nyman S. Periodontal regeneration via selective cell repopulation. J Periodontol 1987;58:546.

40. Gottlow J, Nyman S, Karring T, Lindhe J. New attachment formation as a result of controlled tissue regeneration. J Clin Periodontol 1984;11(8):494.

41. Caffesse RG, Quinones CR. Polypeptide growth factors and attachment proteins in periodontal wound healing and regeneration. Periodontology 2000 1993;1:69.

42. Ripamonti U, Reddi A. Periodontal regeneration: Potential role of bone morphogenetic proteins. J Periodontal Res 1994;29:225.

43. Graves DT, Cochran DL. Periodontal regeneration with polypeptide growth factors. Curr Opin Periodontol 1994:178.

44. Hammarström L, Heijl L, Gestrelius S. Periodontal regeneration in a buccal dehiscence model in monkeys after application of enamel matrix proteins. J Clin Periodontol 1997;24(9):669.

45. Heijl L. Periodontal regeneration with enamel matrix derivative in one human experimental defect. J Clin Periodontol 1997;24(9):693.

46. Heijl L, Heden G, Svardstrom G, Ostgren A. Enamel matrix derivative (Emdogain) in the treatment of intrabony periodontal defects. J Clin Periodontol 1997;24(9):705.

47. Aranjo MG, Lindhe J. GTR treatment of degree III furcation defects following application of enamel matrix proteins. An experimental study in dogs. J Clin Periodontol 1998;25:524.

Safety Testing of Emdogain

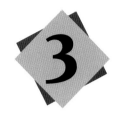

Emdogain contains a sterile protein aggregate from enamel matrix, amelogenin, the precursor of enamel from developing teeth. The hydrophobic protein aggregate is solubilized in a sterile, acidic vehicle solution (propylene glycol alginate) during clinical application. In the physiologic environment of the periodontal lesion, with neutral pH and body temperature, the viscous vehicle solution becomes watery and rapidly leaves the application site, while the protein changes to its natural, aggregated state and forms a matrix on the root surface. A protein layer is absorbed on mineral or collagen surfaces of the dental root and remains for 1 to 2 weeks. The removal takes place via enzymatic degradation, producing only natural amino acids or peptide fragments which are eliminated through the kidneys.[1]

Preclinical Testing

Emdogain has been tested as a new chemical entity with a safety program encompassing single- and multiple-dose studies (intravenous and subcutaneous), local irritation tests (subcutaneous and topical), and in vitro tests for cell toxicity and mutagenicity. No adverse results were found (Biora AB/Data on file).

In addition to these standardized safety studies, Emdogain was also used in studies with monkeys where both effectiveness and safety were followed over time. Rapid and uncomplicated healing was found after applying Emdogain on dentin surfaces after removing buccal bone and cementum of mandibular premolars. No adverse reactions were noticed; instead, the Emdogain-treated defects appeared to exhibit more rapid clinical healing with less recession of the gingiva, and regeneration of the new periodontal attachment apparatus with new acellular cementum, new extrinsic collagen fibers, and new alveolar bone.[2]

Clinical Testing

Immunology

Enamel matrix proteins are expected to be recognized as "self" by the human immune system, because everyone is exposed to them during tooth development in early childhood. The protein in Emdogain is of porcine origin with very high homogeneity to the human amelogenins. Emdogain is purified through a number of processing steps, including solvent and heat treatment, ultrafiltration, sterile filtration, and freeze drying.

One clinical study with Emdogain was performed to test for clinical hypersensitivity, especially type I, the immediate allergic response mediated by IgE. In total, 107 patients had two periodontal surgeries using Emdogain, with the procedures performed 2 to 6 weeks apart. Blood samples were taken either before and after surgery or only after one or two treatments, and compared to samples from a nonexposed control group of 92 blood donors. None of the samples from treated patients indicated changes from the control group. This was also true for 21 patients in the control group who were determined allergy-prone by atopy screening (Phadiatop test); that is, there were no raised titers of any Emdogain-reactive antibodies.[3]

Ten occupationally exposed employees from the laboratories where Emdogain was developed and produced were tested for type IV sensitization by using skin tests with several concentrations of Emdogain and comparing results to negative (buffer) and positive (histamine) controls. No reactions were seen either immediately or within the 48 hours following testing. One year later the same employees volunteered for a challenge injection of Emdogain protein, and blood samples were taken before and a month after this injection. The result was again unchanged; no immunoresponse was elicited.[3]

Postsurgical experiences

All clinical studies with Emdogain have included active questioning of patients for subjective adverse reactions and have required dentists to note any objective reactions. Comparisons in clinical studies between the test surgeries with Emdogain and identical control surgeries without Emdogain showed no differences in type or frequency of common procedure-related experiences such as root sensitivity, mucosal irritation, and so on. When certain antibiotics were used, well-known side effects (eg, skin reactions and gastrointestinal problems) were detected.[3,4]

Postmarketing Surveillance

Emdogain is approved and marketed in Europe, North America, and Japan. Postmarketing surveillance programs are in progress in these markets. By June 1998, about 35,000 treatments had been performed worldwide. No serious adverse events or adverse experiences not commonly associated with periodontal surgery per se had been recorded.

Swedish patients who had been treated at least twice with Emdogain were invited to participate in a skin test of the type previously used in occupationally exposed subjects. Batch EMD 4121 was dissolved and diluted in cold sterile saline with 0.3% human serum albumin (Pharmagen, Pharmacia-Upjohn) to final concentrations of 10 mg/mL, 1.0 mg/mL, and 0.1 mg/mL). A drop of each of these dilutions was placed on the inside of the volar aspect of the left forearm. The point of a lancet was then pressed into the superficial layer of the skin for 1 second. A lancet pretreated with histamine hydrochloride (Soluprick, ALK) was used as a positive control. Immediate wheal reaction was examined after 5, 10, 15, 20, and 30 minutes and registered for comparison to the controls. The histamine and saline controls were measured after 15 minutes, and the diameter of the wheal was noted in the protocol. After 6 and 24 hours, the test area was reexamined for any dose-dependent late cutaneous reactions.

Thirty-seven patients were tested: 31 after two separate Emdogain treatments, 5 after three to four surgeries with Emdogain, and 1 after five such surgeries over a period of 6 months. In the skin test, no instances of immediate or late wheal development were recorded for any patient at any of the Emdogain protein dilutions. A wheal was seen after histamine exposure only (positive control). The uneventful result confirms previous studies with skin tests and immunoassays in which no reactions were found. Because all patients had received two to five treatments with Emdogain, it further supports the conclusion that Emdogain has very low, if any, sensitizing potential.

Summary

As of June 1998, 35,000 treatments with Emdogain had not revealed any adverse experiences other than those commonly found with any type of periodontal surgery, such as pain and swelling. On the contrary, several patients and dentists have reported that the early healing period is quicker and less eventful than with conventional surgery. These statements are now being investigated by new controlled studies.

References

1. Gestrelius S, Andersson C, Johansson A-C, Persson E, Brodin A, Rydhag L, Hammarström L. Formulation of enamel matrix derivative for surface coating. Kinetics and cell colonization. J Clin Periodontol 1997;24:678.

2. Hammarström L, Heijl L, Gestrelius S. Periodontal regeneration in a buccal dehiscence model in monkeys after application of enamel matrix proteins. J Clin Periodontol 1997;24:669.

3. Zetterstrom O, Andersson C, Eriksson L, et al. Clinical safety of enamel matrix derivative (Emdogain) in the treatment of periodontal defects. J Clin Periodontol 1997;24:697.

4. Heijl L, Heden G, Svardstrom G, Ostgren A. Enamel matrix derivative (Emdogain) in the treatment of intrabony periodontal defects. J Clin Periodontol 1997;24:705.

Patient Selection

The patient with the fewest local and systemic risk factors has the best prognosis following therapy for regeneration. The following steps, described in this chapter, outline how to address risk factors and provide more predictable results:

1. Clinical and radiographic examination
2. Identification of risk factors
3. Development of a treatment plan (informed consent)
4. Therapy
5. Maintenance

Clinical and Radiographic Examination

Initial data including a medical and dental history, radiographs of the affected areas, areas of restorative need, periodontal probing depths, gingival recession, endodontic concerns, and tooth mobility should be collected. Details of these procedures are available elsewhere.[1]

Identification of Risk Factors

Local

Any areas that harbor bacteria are important local risk factors. These include restorations that have overhangs, orthodontic appliances that create plaque traps, and periodontal pockets. Another major local risk factor is the degree of the patient's compliance to suggested oral hygiene. In general, the better the personal plaque control, the better the long-term outlook for the dentition. The last major local risk factor is the patient's compliance to suggested maintenance following regenerative procedures; again, in general, the better the compliance, the fewer teeth will be lost.

Systemic

A number of systemic factors can affect the outcome of regeneration. The three that are often encountered and have profound effects on the longevity of the dentition are a history of smoking, diabetes, and the genotype status for the Interleukin-1 (IL-1) gene. This last factor has been linked to premature tooth loss from adult forms of periodontitis.[2] When a patient is a smoker and positive for the IL-1 genotype, the risk of tooth loss is increased substantially (Fig 4-1).[3]

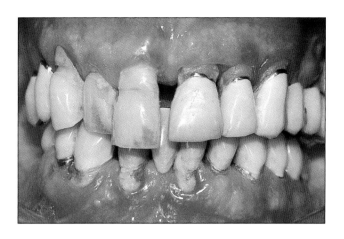

Fig 4-1 This patient was never able to achieve an adequate level of oral hygiene to remove enough bacterial plaque to attain a steady state of periodontal health. He is genotype positive for the IL-1 geno and a smoker; he was not a surgical candidate. Five years after this photograph, his teeth were removed as a result of continued inflammation.

Development of a Treatment Plan (Informed Consent)

After any needed consultations with other dentists and physicians, treatment plans ranging from no treatment through all the possible therapies are presented to the patient. The patient should be informed of the pros and cons of each proposed procedure and given one or two plans that the therapist and his or her group consider optimal. The patient should be given enough information on the various approaches to allow him or her to provide informed consent.

The patient also should be informed at this stage that the more local and systemic risk factors that can be reduced or eliminated, the better the prognosis. In general, the less a patient smokes and the better the control of any diabetes, the better the prognosis. The same is true for compliance with suggested oral hygiene and maintenance procedures (Fig 4-2). Once this stage has been completed, treatment can proceed.

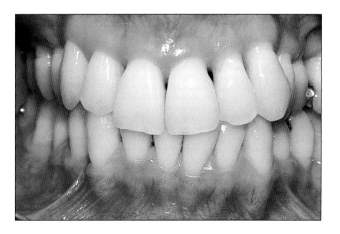

Fig 4-2 Twenty-one years after active treatment (including surgery) for severe periodontitis, this patient has lost no teeth. She is genotype negative for the IL-1 gene, stopped smoking when treatment began, and complied with suggestions for oral hygiene and maintenance care.

Therapy

Before the clinician considers a patient as a surgical candidate, several criteria must be met. The patient must have a level of systemic health that will not negatively affect the surgical outcome. Next, he or she must enter into surgery after acquiring sufficient knowledge to provide his or her informed consent. The level of the patient's oral hygiene should be adequate to sustain a healthy state during initial healing and beyond.

In most cases, the patient will have received and responded unfavorably to closed subgingival scaling and root planing in the areas of proposed surgical intervention. Other forms of initial nonsurgical care also may be warranted. Interventions may include, but not be limited to, modification of risk factors such as diabetes and smoking[4]; control of parafunctional habits such as bruxing[5]; other appropriate therapy to eliminate plaque retentive areas such as restorative margins with overhangs; appropriate methods to reposition the teeth such as orthodontic therapy; and therapy for endodontic lesions where indicated. It is often appropriate to remove teeth slated for extraction during this phase of treatment.

Following the initial, nonsurgical phase of therapy, a reevaluation of treatment is performed. At this evaluation, the same parameters gathered at the initial examination are obtained and compared using the first visit as a baseline. If the IL-1 status has been determined previously, this does not need to be repeated, because genotype status does not change.

If the patient has adequate oral hygiene but there are persistent signs of clinical inflammation where accumulated subgingival tooth-borne debris was successfully removed (usually from nonfurcated teeth), additional diagnostics are needed before further treatment is performed.[6,7] Such diagnostics usually include genotype testing for the IL-1 polymorphism (if this has not been performed previously) and often bacterial sampling and antibiotic specificity testing. If antibiotics are to be used, once they have been identified, intervention can be provided as dictated by the depth and location of the pocket and by the anatomy of the tooth.

Patients who test negative for the IL-1 gene and have signs of clinical inflammation in areas suspected of calculus retention following closed subgingival scaling and root planing, where pathologically deepened pockets are associated with such signs following initial therapy, can often benefit from additional rounds of closed subgingival scaling and root planing.

If these additional rounds fail to halt the disease process, surgery is recommended, because it can provide access for more effective removal of tooth-borne materials. In probing depths of 5 mm or greater, the chances of leaving calculus and tooth-borne bacteria outweigh the chances for removing it when using closed subgingival scaling and root planing.[8,9] However, surgery has been shown to increase the probability of removal of tooth-borne accretions, especially when performed by an experienced operator.[10,11] Removal of these materials increases the chances of forming a steady state between the bacteria and the body by reducing the ecologic niches available to the bacteria and making personal oral hygiene more effective.

Patients who test positive for the IL-1 gene and have probing depths of greater than 5 mm after initial nonsurgical therapy associated with clinical signs of inflammation are at additional risk for future attachment loss compared with genotype-negative individuals presenting with the same clinical parameters.

Genotype-positive patients are more likely to benefit from surgical procedures to reduce probing depths, the rationale being that more pathogenic bacteria are found in deeper pockets and that individuals who are genotype positive are more likely to experience attachment loss as a result compared to those patients who are genotype negative. Thus, by reducing the niches that favor the more aggressive bacteria, it is less likely that future attachment loss will occur.

In some forms of early onset periodontitis, surgery appears necessary to eliminate some of the bacteria closely associated with the disease. In some young adults with severe generalized periodontitis, surgery was needed to eliminate *Actinobacillus actinomycetemcomitans*.[12] Similar results were seen in some patients who experienced rapid attachment loss.[7] Given the tendency of these diseases to recur, surgical procedures that reduce the bacteria or their niches can prove helpful in controlling the disease process.

Maintenance

Several long-term studies done in university settings have shown no difference between the effects of closed subgingival scaling and root planing and those of periodontal surgery.[13-15] The conclusions of these published studies have little relevance to the average patient in the average dental practice. To be included in these studies, patients were required to stay on supportive periodontal treatment (SPT), which plays a major role in the continued stability of deeper probing depths and in preventing recurrence of disease.[16-19]

Unfortunately, the vast majority of patients in private practice do not comply with suggested SPT intervals.[18,20-24] These patients therefore do not benefit from timely professional procedures that could clean out potentially pathologic pockets. However, pocket reduction surgery can provide patients with adequate oral hygiene better access for personal oral hygiene and therefore less potential for disease recurrence for those who are erratically compliant or noncompliant to SPT.

Additional information on patient selection can be found in chapter 5.

References

1. Wilson T, Kornman K. Fundamentals of Periodontics. Chicago: Quintessence, 1996:564.

2. Kornman K, Crane A, Wang H-Y, et al. The Interleukin-1 genotype as a severity factor in adult periodontal disease. J Clin Periodontol 1997;24:72.

3. McGuire MK and Nunn ME. Prognosis versus actual outcome. IV. The effectiveness of clinical parameters and IL-1 genotype in accurately predicting prognosis and tooth survival. J Periodontol (in press).

4. Rosenberg E, Cutler S. The effect of cigarette smoking on the long-term success of guided tissue regeneration: A preliminary study. Ann R Australas Coll Dent Surg 1994;12:89.

5. Burgett F, Ramfjord S, Nissle R, Morrison E, Charberneau T, Caffesse R. A randomized trial of occlusal adjustment in the tratment of periodontitis patients. J Clin Periodontol 1992;19:381.

6. Gordon J, Walkert D. Current status of systemic antibiotic usage in destructive periodontal disease. J Periodontol 1993;64(8 suppl):760.

7. Rosenberg E, Torosian J, Hammond B, Cutler S. Routine anaerobic bacterial culture and systemic antibiotic usage in the treatment of adult periodontitis: A 6-year longitudinal study. Int J Periodontics Restorative Dent 1993;13(3):213.

8. Waerhaug J. Healing of the dento-epithelial junction following subgingival plaque control. II. As observed on extracted teeth. J Periodontol 1978;49(3):119.

9. Stambaugh RV, Dragoo M, Smith DM, Carasal L. The limits of subgingival scaling. Int J Periodontics Restorative Dent 1981;1(5):30.

10. Caffesse RG, Sweeney PL, Smith BA. Scaling and root planing with and without periodontal flap surgery. J Clin Periodontol 1986;13(13):205.

11. Brayer WK, Mellonig JT, Dunlap RM, Marinak KW, Carson RE. Scaling and root planing effectiveness: The effect of root surface access and operator experience. J Periodontol 1989;60(1):67.

12. Gunsolley J, Zambon J, Mellott C, Brooks C, Kaugars C. Periodontal therapy in young adults with severe generalized periodontitis. J Periodontol 1994;65(3):268.

13. Kaldahl WB, Kalkwarf KL, Patil KD, Dyer JK, Bates RE. Evaluation of four modalities of periodontal therapy. Mean probing depth, probing attachment level and recession changes. J Periodontol 1988;59(12):783.

14. Ramfjord S, Caffesse R, Morrison E, et al. Four modalities of periodontal treatment compared over five years. J Periodontal Res 1987;22(3):222.

15. Pihlström B, Oliphant T, McHugh R. Molar and nonmolar teeth compared over 6 1/2 years following two methods of periodontal therapy. J Periodontol 1984;55(9):499.

16. Wilson TG, Glover ME, Malik AK, Schoen JA, Dorsett D. Tooth loss in maintenance patients in a private periodontal practice. J Periodontol 1987;58(4):231.

17. Galgut P. Compliance with maintenance therapy after periodontal treatment. Dent Health (London) 1991;30(6):3.

18. Checchi L, Pelliccioni G, Gatto M, Kelescian L. Patient compliance with maintenance therapy in an Italian periodontal practice. J Clin Periodontol 1994;21(5):309.

19. Bostanci H, Arpack M. Long-term evaluation of surgical periodontal treatment with and without maintenance care. J Nihon Univ Sch Dent 1991;33:152.

20. Wilson TG, Glover ME, Schoen J, Baus C, Jacobs T. Compliance with maintenance therapy in a private periodontal practice. J Periodontol 1984;55(8):468.

21. Wilson T, Hale S, Temple R. The results of efforts to improve compliance with supportive periodontal treatment in a private practice. J Periodontol 1993;64(4):311.

22. Tan A, Powell R, Seymour G. Patient attendance. Compliance in periodontal therapy. Aust Dent J 1992;37(6):467.

23. Galgut P. Compliance with maintenance therapy after periodontal treatment. Dent Health (London) 1992;30(6):3.

24. Mendoza A, Newcomb G, Nixon K. Compliance with supportive periodontal therapy. J Periodontol 1991;62:731.

Surgical Therapy Using Enamel Matrix Proteins

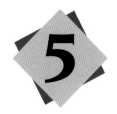

5

This chapter details the selection of periodontal defects that will best respond to the use of enamel matrix proteins. Root preparation procedures and details of the specific use of Emdogain also are covered. Patient selection was discussed in chapter 4. Patients with no systemic risk factors or with factors that can be eliminated are better surgical candidates. Smoking, being positive for the Interleukin-1 (IL-1) genotype, and having diabetes are significant negative systemic risk factors. Smoking can be eliminated and diabetes can often be controlled, thus improving the prognosis, but the IL-1 genotype cannot be changed. In general, the better the patient's oral hygiene and the better his or her compliance to suggested supportive periodontal therapy (maintenance) visits, the better the prognosis.

Selection of Appropriate Surgical Sites

The more carefully one selects bony defects for treatment, the greater the likelihood of success. It is advantageous to remove any tooth-borne areas that favor plaque retention before surgery begins. In general, a tooth with less mobility fares better than a similar tooth having greater mobility. Parafunctional habits are best controlled before surgery begins, as are active endodontic lesions. The patient whose oral cavity is adequate to allow cleaning and preparation of the defect has a better prognosis.

Enamel matrix proteins were originally designed for use in areas that have severe bone loss resulting from periodontitis. It is suggested that the surgeon who is unfamiliar with the use of these materials initially use them in narrow, three-wall bony defects that do not involve furcations (Figs 5-1a to 5-1d). This will give the clinician a chance to gain experience with the product and site preparation.

Figs 5-1a to 5-1t A 33-year-old woman had been diagnosed with severe generalized adult periodontitis. She had good oral hygiene and no systematic risk factors. Following initial nonsurgical periodontal therapy, she was deemed a good candidate for surgery.

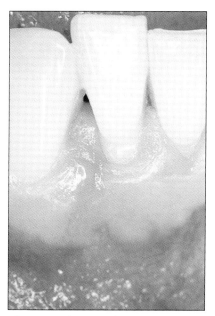

Fig 5-1a Photograph taken prior to treatment.

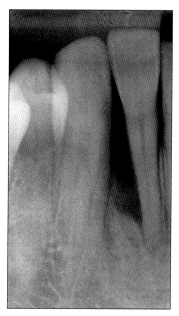

Fig 5-1b Radiograph of the teeth in Fig 5-1a.

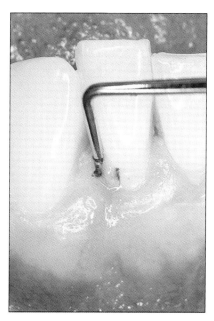

Fig 5-1c Initial probing depths on the distal apect of this mandibular lateral incisor measured 9 mm.

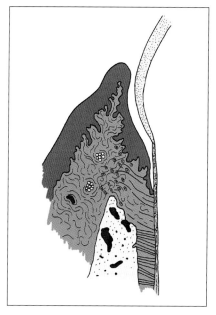

Fig 5-1d Attachment loss is accompanied by hypermineralization of the root surface.

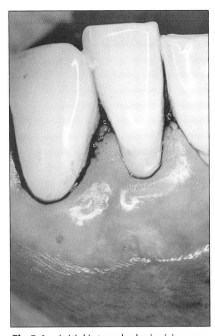

Fig 5-1e Initial intrasulcular incisions are designed to retain as much soft tissue as possible while eliminating the maximum amount of sulcular epithelium.

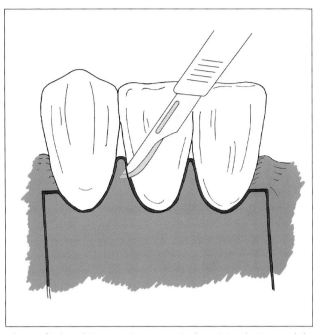

Fig 5-1f The clinician tries to retain keratinized tissue while removing as much of the junctional epithelium as possible with the incision.

Surgical Procedure

Incisions are made that will allow primary closure following surgery (Figs 5-1e and 5-1f). Full-thickness flaps are raised using vertical incisions where appropriate. Once the extent of the defect has been analyzed and the decision to use Emdogain has been made, the material is mixed (or the premixed syringe is removed from refrigeration). When the material is delivered in two separate bottles, the vehicle propylene glycol alginate (PGA) is put into the bottle with the freeze-dried enamel matrix proteins. Once mixed, the material should be used within 2 hours because it tends to harden after this amount of time.

During this period, the surgeon mechanically cleans the root surface using sonic, ultrasonic, hand, or rotary instruments or combinations thereof (Figs 5-1g to 5-1j). The defect itself is thoroughly debrided to remove all the granulation tissue possible.

Next, the smear layer is cleaned from the root surface with neutrally buffered ethylenediaminetetraacetic acid (EDTA) for 2 minutes (Figs 5-1k to 5-1n). (A later section in this chapter explains the rationale for using EDTA for this step.) The assistant irrigates the root surface with large quantities of sterile water or sterile saline. At the same time, high vacuum suction is applied.

The needle of the syringe containing the Emdogain is then placed on the root surface at the bottom of the bony defect. It is critical for the Emdogain to be the first protein that touches the root surface. This is accomplished by the assistant discontinuing the water spray, then slowly removing the suction as the Emdogain is injected onto the root surface in the bony defect (Figs 5-1o and 5-1p). The area is closed as soon as possible (Figs 5-1q and 5-1r).

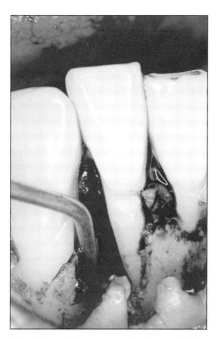

Fig 5-1g Following reflection of full-thickness mucoperiosteal flaps, judicious removal of all granulation tissue and thorough scaling and root planing are performed.

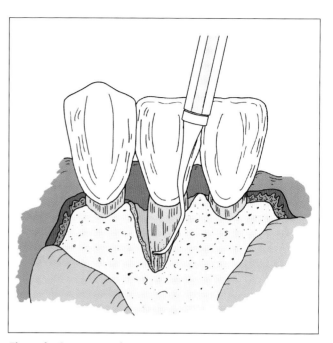

Fig 5-1h Curettes or ultrasonic, sonic, or rotary instruments can be used to remove calculus and other bacterial products from the root surface.

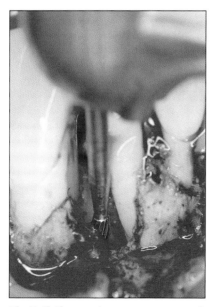

Fig 5-1i If rotary instruments are used, minimal amounts of tooth surface need to be removed.

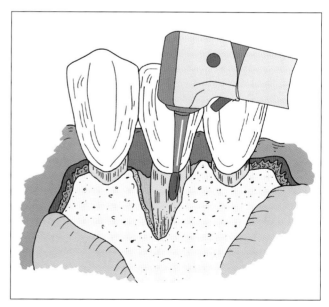

Fig 5-1j The finishing bur is used at slow speeds.

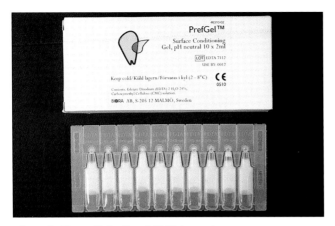

Fig 5-1k Neutrally buffered EDTA is used.

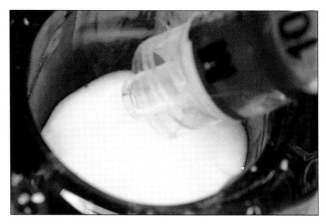

Fig 5-1l The EDTA is drawn up into a syringe.

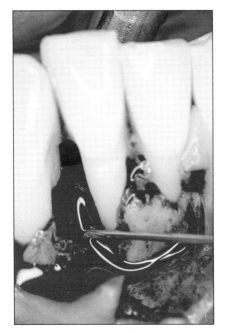

Fig 5-1m A blunt needle is placed on the syringe containing the EDTA, and the material is expressed onto the tooth. It is left in place for 2 minutes.

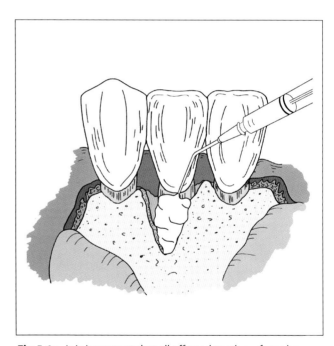

Fig 5-1n It is important that all affected tooth surfaces be covered with EDTA.

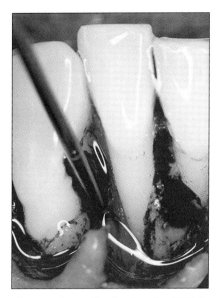

Fig 5-1o Immediately after the EDTA is thoroughly rinsed from the tooth, the Emdogain is expressed onto the surface starting at the base of the bony defect.

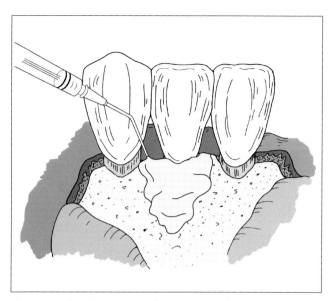

Fig 5-1p The first protein that touches the root should be Emdogain, not blood or saliva.

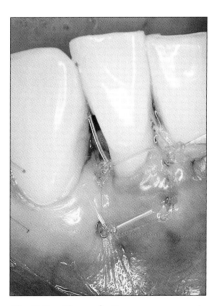

Fig 5-1q The soft tissues are repositioned with nonabsorbable or slowly absorptive sutures.

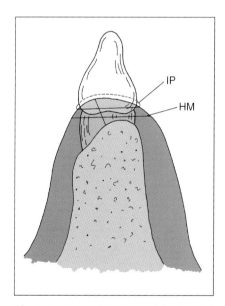

Fig 5-1r A combination of horizontal mattress (HM) and interproximal sutures (IP) are used to achieve primary closure.

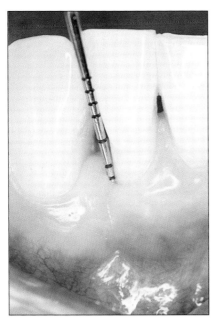

Fig 5-1s The surgical area 16 months following surgery. Compare to Fig 5-1c.

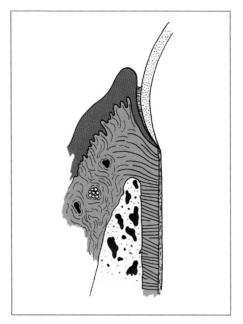

Fig 5-1t The goal is a clinically stable periodontium and regeneration of new cementum, periodontal ligament, and bone.

Following closure, a shift in the pH and temperature occurs that causes the Emdogain to precipitate as an aggregate on the root surface. Once it has precipitated, it becomes insoluble. The area is sutured with material that will cause minimal irritation, such as a monofilament suture. This ensures that the flap remains stable. The patient is then instructed in postoperative care (see chapter 6).

At the first postoperative visit, usually 7 to 10 days after surgery, loose sutures and any debris are removed and the patient is reminded to continue to use a chlorhexidine rinse twice daily. The patient is seen as often as needed to keep the surgical site free of inflammation. After six weeks, normal oral hygiene can be resumed. The desired clinical end result is a shallow sulcus without signs of inflammation (Fig 5-1s). The goal of the surgery is regeneration of the lost periodontal attachment (Fig 5-1t).

Box 5-1 shows the important steps in achieving predictable, successful outcomes for this procedure.

Box 5-1 Keys to Successful Surgical Outcomes

- Make incisions that allow primary closure of the flaps.
- Clean the root surface thoroughly.
- Remove the resulting smear layer.
- Control bleeding in the defect to ensure that the enamel matrix protein touches the root surface before blood or saliva.
- Close the flaps as soon as possible following application of the enamel matrix protein.
- Stabilize the wound. This is usually accomplished with sutures that do not resorb or resorb over several weeks.
- Ensure that the tooth receiving the enamel matrix proteins is stable and that occlusal interferences are removed before or during surgery (optimal situation).
- Provide the patient with the means to successfully remove newly forming dental plaque during healing. Twice daily chlorhexidine rinses are optimal for most patients.
- Monitor the patient frequently during the postoperative phase for adequate bacterial plaque removal and for any developing occlusal interferences.

Removal of the Smear Layer

When teeth lose attachment, previously anchored fibers of gingival connective tissue and of the periodontal ligament become infiltrated with inflammatory cells and lose collagen. This is caused by bacteria and their products[1] and results in a hypermineralized, bacterial infestation on the root surface that precludes regeneration by inhibiting attachment of new cells.[2] To enhance the probability for regeneration, it has been suggested that the root surface be cleansed of these bacteria and their by-products.[3] Numerous mechanical methods are available to accomplish this removal, and all inevitably result in a residue of highly calcified material laden with bacteria and its by-products being spread over the root. This residue is called the "smear layer"[4] and is found regardless of the manner in which the tooth is cleaned.[4–7]

A debate has arisen concerning whether or not regeneration is accelerated by removal of the smear layer and how it is best removed if the clinician decides to do so. The case for removal is strengthened by an ultrastructural study that concluded that the first step toward regeneration in cats was characterized by surface demineralization of apatite crystal on the root surface.[5] Topical application of acids to the root surface demineralizes the surface layer;[6] therefore, it has been suggested that this may facilitate the attachment of a postoperative fibrin clot. This clot is important because it retards apical migration of the epithelium, giving the cells that are necessary for regeneration more time to migrate.[7] This process also exposes collagen fibrils that may enhance fibroblast attachment and growth[8] and allow splicing of newly synthesized collagen to the existing fibrils.[9]

A number of materials have been used to remove the smear layer, including citric acid,[10] tetracycline hydrochloride,[11] EDTA,[12] phosphoric acid,[13] maleic acid,[14] methylene blue,[15] and lactic acid.[16] Those most commonly used are citric acid, tetracycline hydrochloride, and phosphoric acid, but interest in EDTA is growing and it is the subject of several studies.

Citric Acid

Citric acid was suggested for smear layer removal by Register[17] in 1973 and has been studied extensively. This material has been shown to remove smear layer,[15,18–22] but reports vary on its efficacy in gaining new attachment. Although some studies have reported improvement in connective tissue attachment, cementogenesis, and regeneration,[6,22–29] others have not.[30–36] This variation in efficacy may be explained by the different concentrations of acid used or by different methods of application.[15,18,19,22,37]

Tetracycline Hydrochloride

Tetracycline hydrochloride has also been found to be effective for removing smear layer.[11,38–42] This material has been shown to positively influence fibroblast attachment and fibronectin binding.[43–50] Various types of tetracyclines have been suggested, but tetracycline hydrochloride, used for at least 30 seconds, has proven most effective in removing smear layer and opening dentinal tubules.[42]

The solution is prepared by adding 1 standard mL of sterile water to the contents of each capsule, then thoroughly mixing the two. The material is applied with light pressure using a sterile cotton pellet.[42] Another study suggests a 4-minute application of a 10 mg/mL solution is most effective in producing the greatest number of available collagen fibers.[51]

Phosphoric Acid

Phosphoric acid has been used in restorative dentistry for smear layer removal prior to bonding techniques and in endodontic therapy for removal of smear layer formed by instrumentation of the canals.[21] It has been shown to be effective in concentrations ranging from 10% to 37%[14,52] and with various thickeners,[53] although the 37% solution produces rougher collagen tags in the deeper parts of the affected area.[54]

Ethylenediaminetetraacetic Acid

This acid has been used in a nonbuffered form for restorative dentistry,[55] to enhance adhesion of restorative materials to enamel and dentin surfaces, and for endodontic therapy.[51,55] A neutrally buffered form has recently been suggested for use in periodontal regeneration.[56] Whereas nonbuffered acids remove smear layer because of low pH, EDTA acts as a chelating agent. A chelating agent is a material combined with a metal in weakly dissociated complexes in which the metal is part of a molecular ring structure.[56] Chelating agents are divalent cations such as Ca^{2+}, Mg^{2+}, Fe^{2+}, and Pb^{2+} at neutral pH. It has been shown that pHs that are not close to neutral inhibit periodontal ligament fibroblasts.[57] Thus, it is suggested that neutrally buffered EDTA will reduce the probability that the soft tissues of the periodontium will be damaged. This means that the cells found in the periodontal ligament and in the vicinity of the alveolar bone will be available when needed to proliferate on the previously diseased root surface, thereby initiating regeneration.

Ethylenediaminetetraacetic acid has been shown to be effective in removing the smear layer and exposing the collagen fibrils without harming the progenitor cells. One study compared citric acid (pH 1.0), EDTA (pH 7.0), and phosphoric acid (pH 1.0) in vitro on extracted monkey teeth. Both passive and rubbing applications were used for 20 seconds or 3 minutes. Control dentin specimens to which only phosphate buffer was applied were still covered with a smear layer. After passive application, the citric and phosphoric groups had almost smooth interlobular dentin surfaces regardless of treatment time whereas the EDTA groups (20 seconds and 3 minutes) exhibited fibrous structures at both time

intervals (more after 3 minutes). The longer the phosphoric acid was left on the tooth and the more it was rubbed, the more cracks in the tooth surface were seen. In contrast, the EDTA-treated surfaces had a dense fibrous surface with no cracks.

The same study had an in vivo component in which the monkey teeth were treated with phosphoric acid or EDTA for 3 minutes, while a control group remained untreated. The teeth were extracted and approximately 2×3 mm of the attachment apparatus was removed; the teeth were reimplanted without splinting. After 14 days of healing, these teeth were removed and prepared for scanning electron microscopy (SEM). Although they were covered with fiber, none of the control teeth showed complete colonization by cells or tissues and the smear layer was still present. None of the phosphoric acid–treated teeth showed complete cellular coverage of the mechanically denuded areas, and there was little sign of migrating or stationary cells. On the other hand, the EDTA-treated surfaces were filled almost completely with fibroblast-like cells on all test teeth. A conclusion of this study was that EDTA promoted cell migration while citric acid and phosphoric acid did not. A 3-minute application of EDTA was suggested.

In another work, it was found that more collagen fibers were exposed when the hypermineralized surface of the diseased tooth was mechanically removed and followed by EDTA placement.[58] The same group of authors investigated the effect of the concentration of EDTA on smear layer removal and collagen exposure.[59] Periodontally involved teeth were extracted and various concentrations of EDTA were placed for 2 minutes, followed by evaluation using SEM. The authors found that concentrations of 15% to 24% EDTA were most effective in removing smear layer and exposing collagen fibers. Another study by this same group found that a 2-minute exposure to 24% neutrally buffered EDTA removed smear layer but resulted in varying degrees of fiber exposure.[60]

Another study looked at the vitality of the periodontal tissues following application of citric acid, phosphoric acid, and neutrally buffered EDTA.[61] Soft-tissue flaps were bathed in the various preparations for 20 seconds and for 3 minutes. Windows were mechanically prepared to remove the periodontal ligament, and the underlying tooth surfaces were treated with various materials. The tissues were incubated and checked for evidence of cellular activity using lactate dehydrogenase activity. Cellular activity was found in the control (saline) and EDTA-treated specimens, but not in the phosphoric acid and citric acid test groups. Phosphoric acid resulted in the greatest demineralization of the root surface but killed cells with an application of only 20 seconds. Citric acid had a less profound effect on demineralization but also killed cells. It should be noted that this effect in vivo may be transient.[62]

The negative effect of low pH acids was further investigated by Blomlof et al.[63] On molars in monkeys, the attachment apparatus was removed with a bur following elevation of full-thickness flaps. Roots were then treated with 37% phosphoric acid for 20 seconds or for 3 minutes. When the teeth were removed 8 weeks later, findings included that those tissues exposed to the acid for 20 seconds healed better than those exposed for 3 minutes, but that both groups experienced reduced healing when compared to controls.

In the last study in the series, EDTA was found to enhance healing when compared to citric acid.[64] After using a surgical technique similar to that described by Blomlof et al,[63] the authors studied monkeys that had no oral hygiene care for 8 weeks following periodontal surgery. They found 10% less failure, as measured by gingival recession and periodontal pocket formation; 10% to 15% more histologic attachment (in the junctional epithelium, connective tissue, and reparative cementum); 20% less length in the junctional epithelium; and 20% more connective tissue on roots etched with EDTA.

Although two of the studies mentioned found that low pH had no negative effect on soft tissue healing,[62,65] it appears that neutrally buffered EDTA removes smear layer and exposes the needed collagen while doing little or no damage to soft tissue.

Therefore, with the information currently available, it appears that removal of smear layer before placement of the enamel matrix proteins is reasonable and that EDTA is a good choice for the removal process.

Possible Applications for Gingival Recession

Denuded areas of the root surface have successfully been covered clinically and regeneration has been demonstrated histologically using enamel matrix proteins. This argues for the use of these proteins in areas of gingival recession. If these materials are chosen to repair areas of esthetic concern where gingival recession has occurred (Figs 5-2a and 5-2b), the steps are similar to those used for bony defects.

Once the decision has been made to treat recession, incisions are made in the same way detailed for periodontal pockets (Figs 5-2c and 5-2d). A full-thickness flap is raised with periosteal scoring and is extended mesiodistally. Vertical incisions may be used to allow the flap to be coronally positioned without tension (Figs 5-2e to 5-2h). This author suggests that the root prominence be removed (Figs 5-2i to 5-2l). The integrity of the pulp should be compromised as little as possible, and the tooth should be reduced until it is flat with the bony housing on the mesial and distal aspects.

The tooth surface is then prepared with neutrally buffered EDTA (Figs 5-2m to 5-2p) and the Emdogain is placed (Figs 5-2q and 5-2r). The flap is placed over the site to allow the enamel matrix proteins to precipitate (Figs 5-2s and 5-2t) while the soft tissue graft is harvested. A subepithelial connective tissue is taken from the palate (Figs 5-2u to 5-2z). The graft is sutured in place (Figs 5-2aa and 5-2bb), the donor site is closed (Figs 5-2cc and 5-2dd), and the flap is sutured over the graft (Figs 5-2ee and 5-2ff). The tissues should heal rapidly (Figs 5-2gg and 5-2hh) and cover the recession (Figs 5-2ii and 5-2jj).

Figs 5-2a to 5-2jj A 25-year-old woman presented with esthetic concerns about the gingival recession on the facial aspect of a maxillary first premolar. The patient also complained of severe sensitivity to cold in the area. There was no bidigital mobility or fremitus.

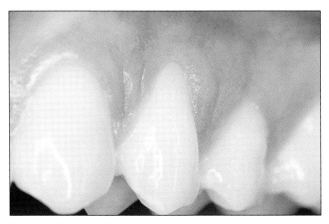

Fig 5-2a Photograph taken prior to treatment.

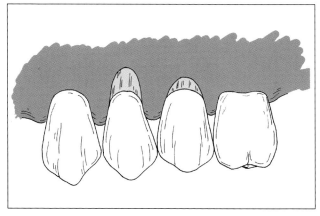

Fig 5-2b The soft tissues showed no signs of clinical inflammation.

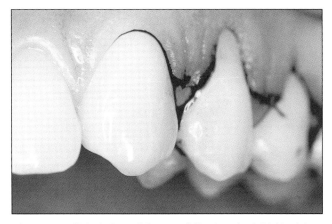

Fig 5-2c A clinical view of the area following the initial incision. An attempt is made to remove the sulcular epithelium.

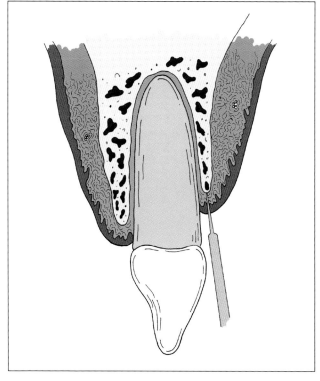

Fig 5-2d The knife blade is slanted toward the alveolar crest.

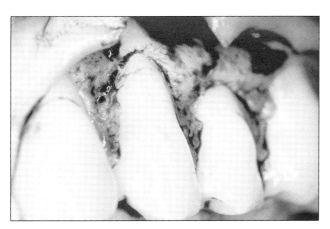

Fig 5-2e A full-thickness mucoperiosteal flap is raised. Vertical incisions are avoided if possible.

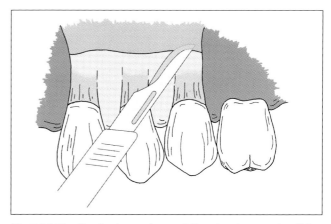

Fig 5-2f The flap is elevated to mobilize the tissue so it will lay passively at the desired position.

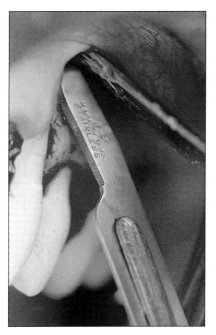

Fig 5-2g In many cases, using a new scalpel blade to dissect the periosteum at the base of the flap will help mobilize the flap.

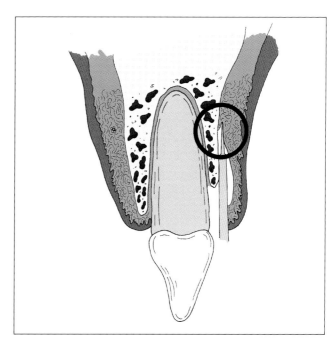

Fig 5-2h Care should be taken to cut through the periosteum but to keep the flap base as thick as possible *(circle)*.

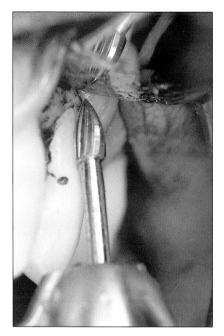

Fig 5-2i The prominence of the tooth on the facial (or lingual) is aspect reduced.

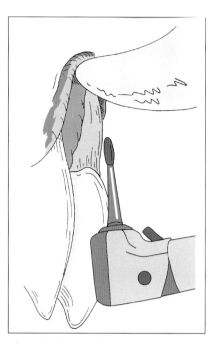

Fig 5-2j The tooth prominence before reduction.

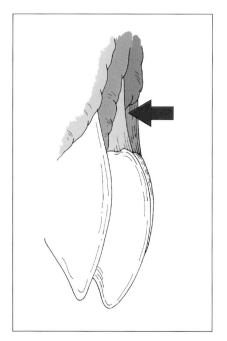

Fig 5-2k During reduction, care should be taken not to compromise the endodontic status of the tooth *(arrow)*.

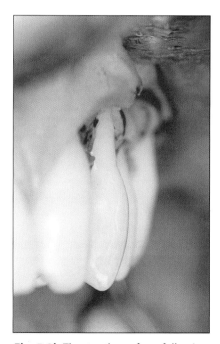

Fig 5-2l The tooth surface following reduction.

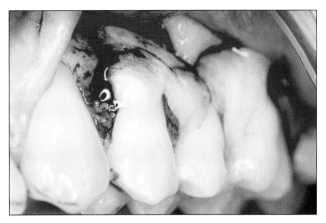

Fig 5-2m Neutrally buffered EDTA is placed on the teeth for 2 minutes.

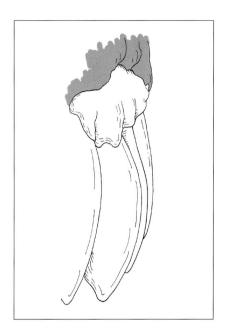

Fig 5-2n Blood does not negatively affect EDTA.

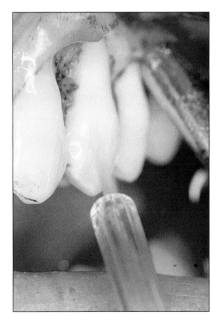

Fig 5-2o The EDTA is thoroughly removed with copious amounts of sterile water and saline.

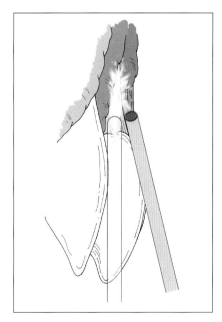

Fig 5-2p Saliva is kept away from the tooth surface.

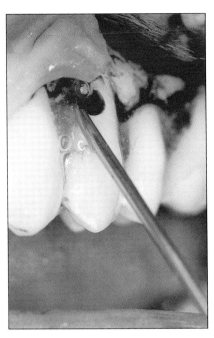

Fig 5-2q The needle of the syringe containing Emdogain is placed at the base of the tooth as the water and suction are withdrawn.

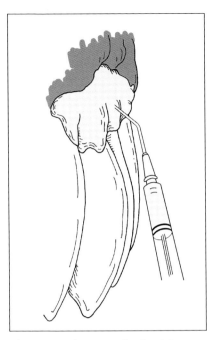

Fig 5-2r At this stage, the tip of the needle containing the Emdogain is placed at the base of the defect.

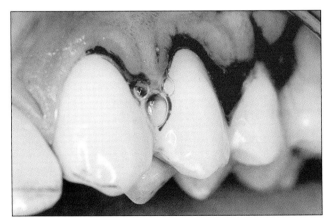

Fig 5-2s The flap is placed over the Emdogain for 1 to 2 minutes to allow the material to precipitate onto the root surface.

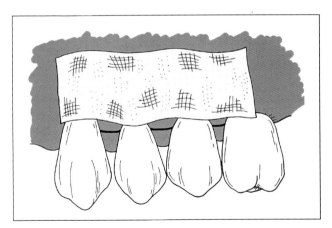

Fig 5-2t Gauze dipped in sterile water or saline can be used to hold the flap in place while the graft is taken.

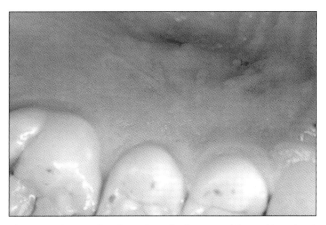

Fig 5-2u Connective tissue is to be harvested from this palatal donor site.

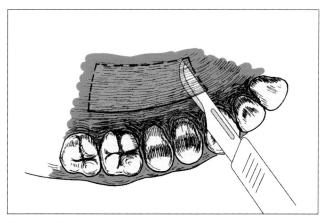

Fig 5-2v The donor site is incised as outlined. The dotted-line area is not cut.

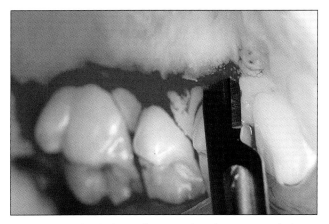

Fig 5-2w A split-thickness flap is made to harvest a graft that is 1 to 1.5 mm thick and large enough to cover the graft site.

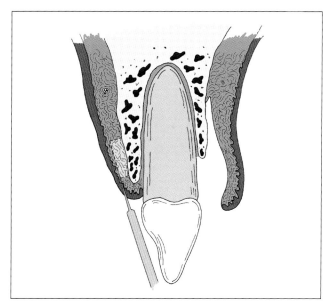

Fig 5-2x A cross-sectional drawing indicates the area of the donor site.

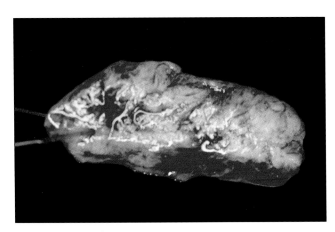

Fig 5-2y The graft.

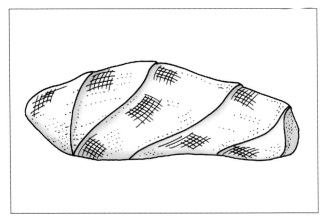

Fig 5-2z The graft should be covered with moistened sterile gauze if it is not immediately sutured in place.

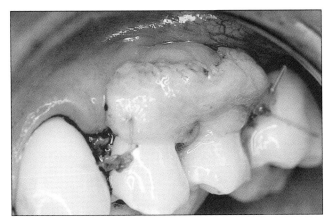

Fig 5-2aa The graft is sutured in place using absorbable sutures such as chromic catgut.

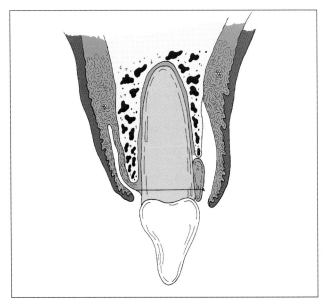

Fig 5-2bb The sutured graft in cross section.

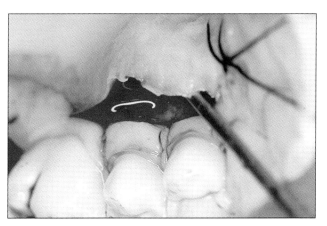

Fig 5-2cc The excess Emdogain is placed in the donor site to aid healing.

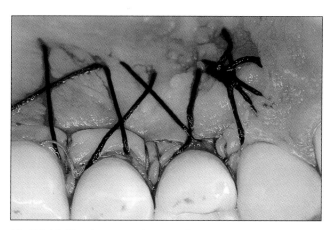

Fig 5-2dd The donor area is sutured.

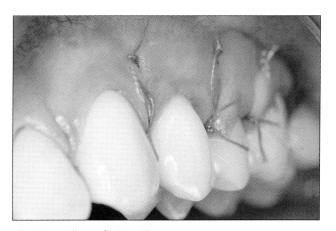

Fig 5-2ee The graft site with oversutures.

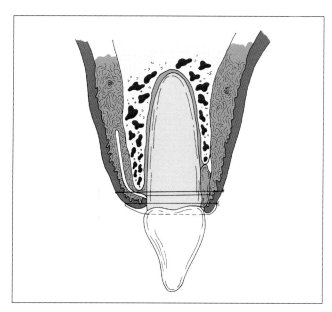

Fig 5-2ff A cross section showing the suturing of the graft and flap.

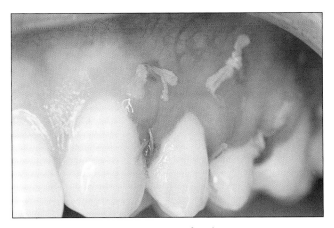

Fig 5-2gg One week postoperative facial view.

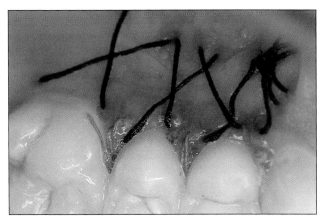

Fig 5-2hh One week postoperative view of the donor site.

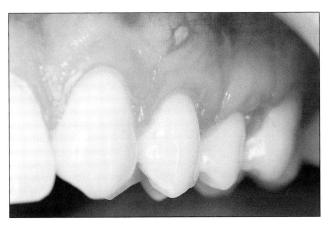

Fig 5-2ii Twelve-month postoperative view.

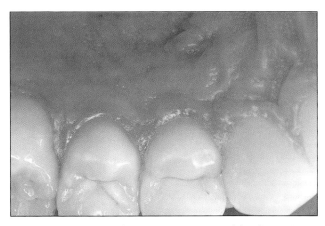

Fig 5-2jj Twelve-month postoperative view of the donor site.

References

1. Hatfield CG, Baujammers A. Cytotoxic effects of periodontally involved surfaces of human teeth. Arch Oral Biol 1971;16:465.

2. Aleo JJ, De Renzis FA, Farber PA. In vitro attachment of human gingival fibroblasts to root surfaces. J Periodontol 1975;46:639.

3. Armitage GC. Biologic basis of scaling and root planing. In: Berkeley, eds. Biologic basis of periodontal maintenance therapy. Praxis: 1980:78.

4. Polson A, Frederick GT, Ladenheim S, Hanes P. The production of a root surface smear layer by instrumentation and its removal by citric acid. J Periodontol 1984;55(8):443.

5. Nalbandian J, Frank RM. Electron microscopic study of the regeneration of cementum and periodontal connective tissue attachment in the cat. J Periodontal Res 1980;13:155.

6. Selvig KA, Ririe CM, Nilveus R, Egelberg J. Fine structure of new connective tissue attachment following acid treatment of experimental furcation pockets in dogs. J Periodontal Res 1981;16:123.

7. Polson AM, Proye MP. Fibrin linkage. A precursor for new attachment. J Periodontol 1983;54:141.

8. Boyko GA, Brunette DM, Melcher AH. Cell attachment to demineralized root surfaces in vitro. J Periodontal Res 1980;15:297.

9. Garret JS, Crigger M, Egelberg J. Effects of citric acid on diseased root surfaces. J Periodontal Res 1978;13:155.

10. Register AA. Bone and cementum induction by dentin, demineralized in situ. J Periodontol 1973;44:49.

11. Labahn TL, Fahrenbach WH, Clark SM, Lie T, Adams DF. Root dentin morphology after different modes of citric acid and tetracycline hydrochloride conditioning. J Periodontol 1992;63:303.

12. Pitaru S, Gray A, Aubin JE, Melcher AH. The influence of the morphological and chemical nature of dental surfaces on the migration, attachment, and orientation of human gingival fibroblasts in vitro. J Periodontal Res 1984;19:408.

13. Leidal TL, Eriksen HM. A scanning electron microscopic study of the effect of various cleansing agents on cavity walls in vitro. Scand J Dent Res 1979;87:443.

14. Mates B, Matson E, Saraceni CH, Palma RG. Effects of acid etching on dentin surface: SEM morphological study. Braz Dent J 1997;8:35.

15. Morgan LA, Baumgartner JC. Demineralization of resected root ends with methylene blue dye. Oral Surg Oral Med Oral Pathol Oral Radiol Endod 1997;84:74.

16. Ayad MF, Farag AM, Rosenstiel SF. A pilot study of lactic acid as an enamel and dentin conditioner. J Prosthet Dent 1996;76:254.

17. Register A, Burdick F. Accelerated reattachment with cementogenesis to dentin, demineralized in situ. II. Defect repair. J Periodontol 1976;47:497.

18. de Araujo F, Issao M, Garcia-Godoy F. A comparison of three resin bonding agents to primary tooth dentin. Pediatr Dent 1997;19(4):253.

19. Chailertvanitkul P, MacKenzie D, Saunders WP. The effect of smear layer on microbial coronal leakage of gutta-percha root fillings. Pediatr Dent 1997;19(4):253.

20. Cagidiaco MC, Davidson CL, Ferrari M. Comparison of in vivo and in vitro demineralized dentin with phosphoric and maleic acid. ASDC J Dent Child 1997;64(1):17.

21. Abitbol T, Scherer W, Santi E, Settembrini L. Root surface biomodification using a dentin bonding conditioner. Periodontal Clin Investig 1996;18(2):27.

22. Higashi T, Okamoto H. The effect of ultrasonic irrigation before and after citric acid treatment on collagen fibril exposure: An in vitro SEM study. J Periodontol 1995;66(10):887.

23. Cole RT, Nilveus R, Ainamo J, Boyle G, Crigger M, Egelberg J. Pilot clinical studies on the effect of topical citric acid application on healing after replaced flap surgery. J Periodontal Res 1981;16:117.

24. Ririe CM, Crigger M, Selvig KA. Healing of periodontal connective tissues following surgical wounding and application of citric acid in dogs. J Periodontal Res 1980;15(3):314.

25. Crigger M, Bogle G, Nilveus R, Egelberg J, Selvig K. The effect of topical citric acid application on the healing of experimental furcation defect in dogs. J Periodontal Res 1978;13:538.

26. Hanes P, Polson A, Ladenheim S. Cell and fiber attachment to demineralized dentin from normal root surfaces. J Periodontol 1985;56:752.

27. Hanes P, Polson A. Cell and fiber attachment to demineralized cementum from normal root surfaces. J Periodontol 1989;60:188.

28. Polson A, Ladenheim S, Hanes P. Cell and fiber attachment to demineralized dentin from periodontitis-affected root surfaces. J Periodontol 1986;57:235.

29. Frank R, Fiore-Donno G, Cimasoni G. Cementogenesis and soft tissue attachment after citric acid treatment in a human. An electric microscopic study. J Periodontol 1983;54:389.

30. Stahl S, Froum S. Human clinical and histologic repair responses following the use of citric acid in periodontal therapy. J Periodontol 1977;48:261.

31. Marks SJ, Mehta N. Lack of effect of citric acid treatment of root surfaces on the formation of new connective tissue. J Clin Periodontol 1986;13:109.

32. Nyman S, Lindhe J, Karring T. Healing following surgical treatment and root demineralization in monkeys with periodontal disease. J Clin Periodontol 1981;8:249.

33. Froum S, Kushner L, Stahl S. Healing responses of human intraosseous lesions following the use of debridement, grafting and citric acid root treatment. I. Clinical and histologic observations six months post-surgery. J Periodontol 1983;54(2):67.

34. Gottlow J, Nyman S, Karring T. Healing following citric acid conditioning of roots implanted into bone and gingival connective tissue. J Periodontol 1984;19:214.

35. Ibbott C, Oles R, Laverty W. Effect of citric acid treatment on autogenous free graft coverage of localized recession. J Periodontol 1985;56:663.

36. Moore JA, Ashley FP, Waterman CA. The effect on healing of the application of citric acid during replaced flap surgery. J Clin Periodontol 1987;14(3):130.

37. Schröeder H. Biological problems of regenerative cementogenesis: Synthesis and attachment of collagenous matrices on growing and established root surface. Int Rev Cytol 1992;142:1.

38. Hanes P, O'Brien N, Garnick J. A morphological comparison of radicular dentin following root planing and treatment with citric acid or tetracycline HCl. J Clin Periodontol 1991;18:660.

39. Lafferty T, Gher M, Gray J. Comparative SEM study on the effect of acid etching with tetracycline HCl or citric acid on instrumented periodontally involved human root surfaces. J Periodontol 1993;64:689.

40. Trombelli L, Scabbia A, Calura G. Nondiseased cementum and dentin root surface following tetracycline hydrochloride conditioning: SEM study of the effects of solution concentration and application time. Int J Periodontics Restorative Dent 1994;14:461.

41. Trombelli L, Scabbia A, Zangari F, Griselli A, Wikesjö U, Calura G. Effect of tetracycline HCl on periodontally affected human root surfaces. J Periodontol 1995;66: 685.

42. Madison JG, Hockett SD. The effects of different tetracyclines on the dentin root surface of instrumented, periodontally involved human teeth: A comparative scanning electron microscope study. J Periodontol 1997; 68(8):739.

43. Terranova V. A biochemical approach to periodontal regeneration—Tetracycline treatment of dentin promoting fibroblast adhesion and growth. J Periodontal Res 1986;21:330.

44. Frantz B, Polson A. Tissue interactions with dentin specimens after demineralization using tetracycline. J Periodontol 1988;59:714.

45. Trombelli L, Schincaglia G, Zangari F, Griselli A, Scabbia A, Calura G. Effects of tetracycline HCl conditioning and fibrin-fibronectin system application in the treatment of buccal gingival recession with guided tissue regeneration. J Periodontol 1995;66:313.

46. Rompen E, Kohl J, Nusgens B, Lapiere C. Kinetic aspects of gingival and periodontal ligament fibroblast attachment to surface-conditioned dentin. J Dent Res 1993;72:607.

47. Somerman M, Foster R, Vorsteg G, Progebin K, Wynn R. Effects of minocycline on fibroblast attachment and spreading. J Periodontol 1988;23:154.

48. Eick J, Wilko R, Anderson C, Sorenson S. Scanning electron microscopy of cut tooth surfaces and identification of debris by use of the electron microscope. J Dent Res 1970;49:1359.

49. Pameijer C, Stallard R, Hiep N. Surface characteristics of teeth following periodontal instrumentation: A scanning electron microscope study. J Periodontol 1972;43:628.

50. Wilkinson R, Maybury J. Scanning electron microscopy of the root surface following instrumentation. J Periodontol 1973;44:559.

51. Barkhordar RA, Hussain MZ, Marshall GW, Watanabe LG. Removal of intracanal smear by doxycycline in vitro. Oral Surg Oral Med Oral Pathol Oral Radiol Endod 1997;84(4):420.

52. DeAraujo FB, Issao M, Garcia-Godoy F. In vivo adhesive interface between resin and dentin. Oper Dent 1995;20(5):204.

53. Perdigao J, Lopes AB, Vanherle G, Tome AR, van Meerbeek B, Lambrechts P. Morphological field emission-SEM study of the effect of six phosphoric acid etching agents on human dentin. Dent Mater 1996;12(4):262.

54. Shimada Y, Takatsu T, Burrow MF, Inokoshi S, Harnirattisai C. In vivo adhesive interface between resin and dentin. Oper Dent 1995;20(5):204.

55. Weiger R, Lost C, Hahn R, Heuchert T. Adhesion of a glass ionomer cement to human radicular dentine. Endod Dent Traumatol 1995;11(5):214.

56. Blömlof J, Lindskog S. Root surface texture and early cell and tissue colonization after different etching modalities. Eur J Oral Sci 1995;103:17.

57. Lengheden A. Influence of pH and calcium on growth and attachment of human fibroblasts in vitro. J Dent Res 1994;102:130.

58. Blömlof J. Root cementum appearance in healthy monkeys and periodontitis-prone patients after different etching modalities. J Clin Periodontol 1996;23:12.

59. Blömlof J, Blömlof L, Lindskog S. Effect of different concentrations of EDTA on smear removal and collagen exposure in periodontitis affected root surfaces. Int J Periodontics Restorative Dent 1997;17:3.

60. Blömlof J, Blömlof L, Lindskog S. Smear layer formed by different root planing modalities and its removal by an EDTA gel preparation. Int J Periodontics Restorative Dent 1997;

61. Blömlof J, Lindskog S. Periodontal tissue-vitality after different etching modalities. J Clin Periodontol 1995;22:464.

62. Seymor G, Romaniuk K, Newcomb G. Effect of citric acid on soft tissue healing in the rat palate. J Clin Periodontol 1983;10:182.

63. Blömlof J, Jansson L, Blömlof L, Lindskog S. Long-time etching at low pH jeopardizes periodontal healing. J Clin Periodontol 1995;22:459.

64. Blömlof J, Jansson L, Blömlof L, Lindskog S. Root surface etching at neutral pH promotes periodontal healing. J Clin Periodontol 1996;23:50.

65. Valenza V, D'Angelo M, Farina-Lipari E, Farina F, Marigotta V. Effects of citric acid on human gingival epithelium. J Periodontol 1987;58:794.

Clinical Application: Case Studies

6

This chapter contains the case reports and clinical photographs of nine patients treated by the author. First, periodontal defects treated with Emdogain alone are described, followed by cases that combined enamel matrix proteins with other materials or that illustrate their use for indications other than infrabony periodontal lesions.

To ensure the greatest potential for success, remember to incorporate the following concepts in therapy.

Review

Patient Selection

The following *systemic risk factors* should be avoided:

- Smoking
- Being positive for the IL-1 genotype
- Having diabetes

The clinician should be able to positively influence the following *local risk factors*:

- The reduction of probing depths to the point that the patient can remove pathogenic bacteria with personal oral hygiene
- The patient's personal oral hygiene
- The patient's compliance to suggested schedules for supportive periodontal therapy (maintenance)
- The removal of impediments, such as poorly fitting dental restorations or the elimination of bacterial plaque

The following *tooth risk factors* should be avoided:

- One- and two-wall bony defects (three-wall defects respond more predictably to regeneration)
- Tooth mobility
- Furcation invasion
- Parafunctional habits (eg, bruxing, clenching)
- Active endodontic lesions

Therapy

The following *preoperative steps* should be taken:

- Any needed consent forms are signed by the patient.
- An antibiotic is prescribed. (optional)
- Ibuprofen (600 mg) is taken 1 hour preoperatively and continued every 6 hours for 2 to 3 days to reduce postoperative discomfort. (optional)
- Any other appropriate medications are taken.

The following *surgical factors* are desirable:

- The surgeon has experience with regeneration techniques.
- The surgeon has adequate access to clean the root and prepare the defect.
- Wound stability is maintained postoperatively.
- The patient complies with suggested postoperative procedures.

The following *postoperative steps* should be taken:

- A narcotic analgesic is used if needed.
- Ice packs are used extraorally over the wound site. They are removed and replaced every 10 minutes for up to 24 hours.
- Twice daily chlorhexidine rinses are started 24 hours following surgery and continued for up to 6 weeks.
- The patient is seen 7 to 10 days postoperatively for follow-up. At each visit, any bacterial plaque or debris is removed carefully from the surgical site.
- Sutures are removed (as needed) at 7 to 14 days.
- The patient does not use normal oral hygiene instruments to clean the surgical wound for 4 to 6 weeks.
- The patient is seen frequently enough to keep the wound site clinically healthy.
- Following healing (usually 2 to 4 months), the patient is placed on a schedule of supportive periodontal therapy (maintenance) every three months or less.
- Probing depths, using normal pressure, are taken 6 months postoperatively.

Case Reports

Case 1 (Figs 6-1a to 6-1e)

This 45-year-old man had been seen sporadically for periodontal maintenance. The probing depths distal to the mandibular right second molar increased over an 8-year period. Once oral hygiene compliance improved, periodontal flap surgery was performed using enamel matrix proteins.

A three-wall bony defect 8 mm in depth was found on the distal aspect of the tooth. Bone loss did not extend to the furcations. Following thorough debridement of the defect and root surface, neutrally buffered EDTA PrefGel (Biora, Malmo) was placed on the root surface for 2 minutes. After thorough rinsing with sterile water, Emdogain was placed on the root before blood or saliva could contaminate the surface.

The area was closed with nonresorbing sutures. The patient took a broad spectrum penicillin 24 hours before the surgery and continued three times daily for 8 days. A chlorhexidine rinse was prescribed for 6 weeks' use.

The patient's compliance to suggested oral hygiene and maintenance was very good, and the probing depth was 3 mm 2 years after therapy. This case is an example of one that could be used to gain experience in handling enamel matrix proteins.

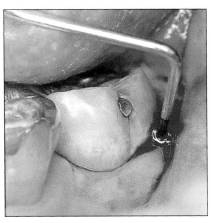

Fig 6-1a A 52-year-old man had received and did not respond to nonsurgical periodontal therapy. There was no bone loss in the furcation on this second molar.

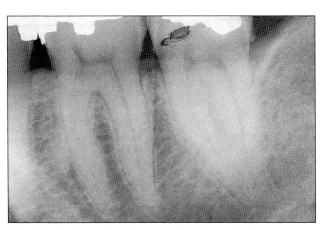

Fig 6-1b Radiograph of the area taken 8 years before surgery.

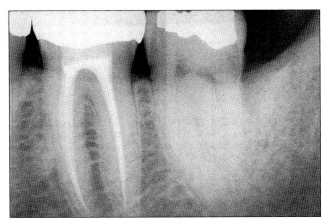

Fig 6-1c Radiograph taken just before surgery. The bony portion of the pocket was 6 mm deep and up to 3 mm wide. No bone loss was found in the furcations.

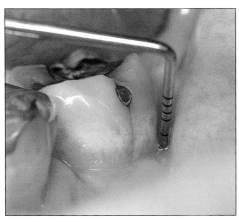

Fig 6-1d The area 16 months postoperatively. The probing depth was 3 mm and the soft tissues were clinically healthy.

Fig 6-1e Radiograph taken 2 years post-operatively.

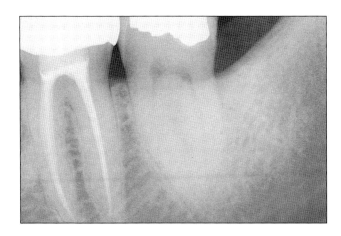

Case 2 (Figs 6-2a to 6-2i)

This clinical presentation and therapy are similar to case 1, but the follow-up radiographs in this case (taken 12 months postoperatively) show less bone deposition than seen in case 1. This may be because the patient had a two-wall, not a three-wall, bony crater; the surgery may not have been performed to the same endpoint; or the enamel matrix proteins were not as effective in this case. It is possible that more bone will be seen radiographically as the postoperative course lengthens.

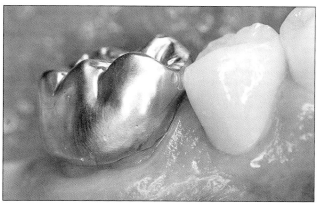

Fig 6-2a A 64-year-old woman presented with a chief complaint of periodic swelling on the mesial apect of the mandibular left first molar. Previous closed subgingival scaling and root planing had not resulted in clinical resolution.

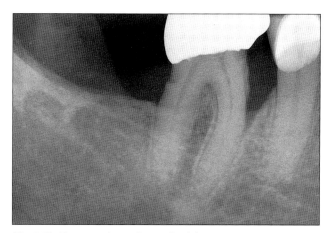

Fig 6-2b Preoperative radiograph of the area.

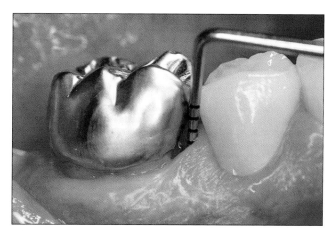

Fig 6-2c The mesial aspect of the tooth had a 7-mm probing depth on the facial aspect and an 8-mm probing depth on the lingual aspect.

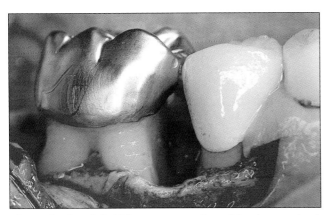

Fig 6-2d When full-thickness mucoperiosteal flaps were raised, a 4- to 5-mm three-wall bony crater was found.

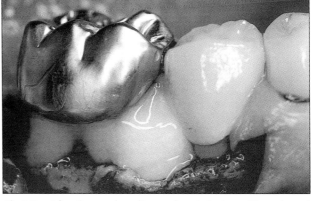

Fig 6-2e After thorough scaling and root planing with sonic and rotary instruments, ethylenediaminetetraacetic acid (EDTA) was placed on the root surface for 2 minutes.

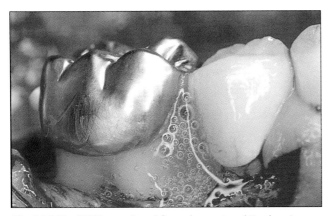

Fig 6-2f The EDTA was rinsed from the root and Emdogain was applied immediately.

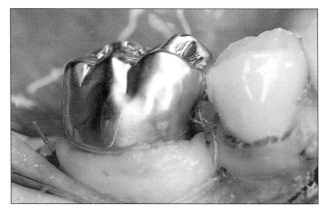

Fig 6-2g The flap was replaced and sutured with a slowly resorbing monofilament suture.

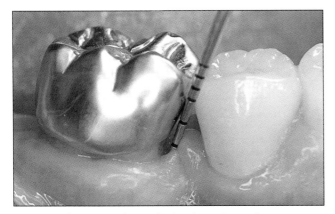

Fig 6-2h The area with a probe in place 12 months postoperatively. Approximately 4 mm of clinical attachment was gained.

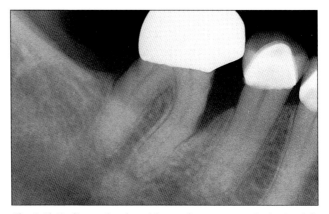

Fig 6-2i Radiograph taken 12 months postoperatively. A minimal amount of increased radiopacity was seen. It may take longer than 1 year for the radiopacity to increase (compare with Fig 6-3f).

Case 3 (Figs 6-3a to 6-3f)

Radiographic response is much more positive in the case of this 56-year-old woman, following surgery with enamel matrix proteins. However, her response to earlier treatment was less positive clinically and radiographically.

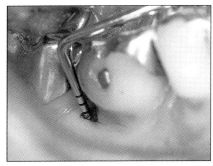

Fig 6-3a This periodontal defect had worsened during the 8 years previous to presentation in spite of two surgical therapies and repeated subgingival scaling and root planing.

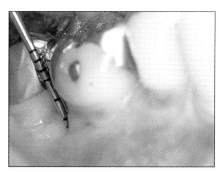

Fig 6-3b Clinical view taken 17 months after that in Fig 6-3a. Probing depths are greatly reduced.

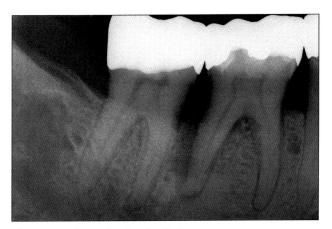

Fig 6-3c Radiograph taken just before surgery.

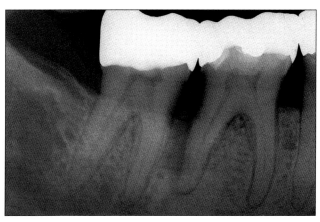

Fig 6-3d Radiograph taken 4 months postoperatively.

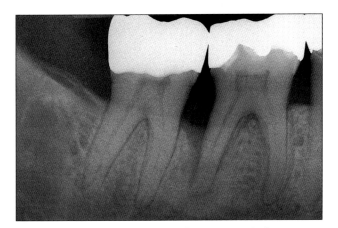

Fig 6-3e Radiograph taken 8 months postoperatively.

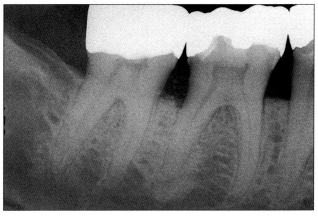

Fig 6-3f Radiograph taken 17 months postoperatively. Note the increased opacity.

Clinical Application: Case Studies

Case 4 (Figs 6-4a to 6-4d)

A 24-year-old man presented with multiple periodontal probing depths of 6 mm or greater. Following surgery with enamel matrix proteins, his probing depths decreased to normal.

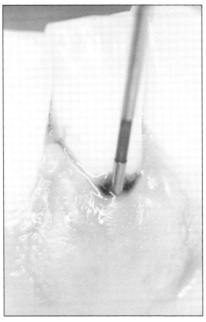

Fig 6-4a This 6-mm defect had not responded to repeated rounds of closed subgingival scaling and root planing.

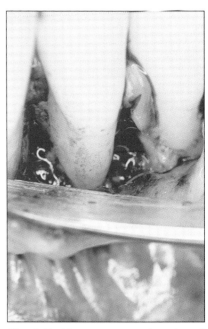

Fig 6-4b The root was planed and treated with EDTA, and Emdogain was placed.

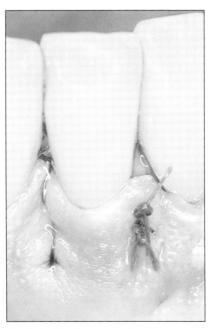

Fig 6-4c The flap was sutured.

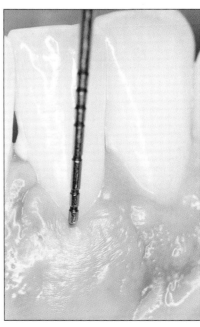

Fig 6-4d The area had a probing depth of 1 mm 18 months postoperatively; 1 mm of gingival recession had occurred.

Case 5 (Figs 6-5a to 6-5d)

A deep bony lesion was found on the mesial surface of the terminal abutment for a three-unit fixed partial denture in a 52-year-old man. A large enamel pearl was found when full-thickness mucoperiosteal flaps were raised. After removal of the pearl and placement of enamel matrix proteins, the flaps were unsupported. Bio-Oss (Osteohealth) was mixed with the remaining enamel matrix proteins and placed into the bony defect to prevent collapse of the flaps. One and a half years later, the probing depth was greatly reduced and the radiographic results substantially improved.

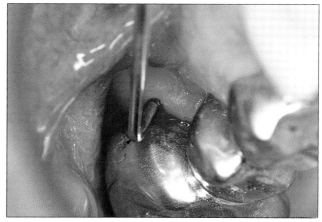

Fig 6-5a A patient presented with a deep periodontal lesion on the terminal abutment for a fixed partial denture.

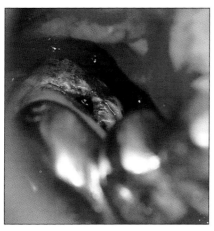

Fig 6-5b A large enamel pearl was found associated with a periodontal defect that approached the apex.

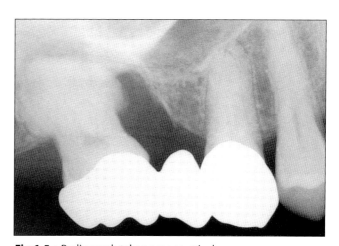

Fig 6-5c Radiograph taken preoperatively.

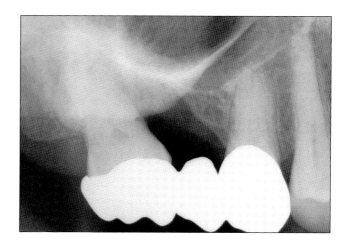

Fig 6-5d Radiograph taken 16 months following the use of Emdogain and Bio-Oss. The probing depth was 5 mm.

Case 6 (Figs 6-6a to 6-6e)

This patient was 45 years old when he presented for periodontal and implant surgery. A one-wall defect was found on the distal aspect of the maxillary left canine. Following placement of enamel matrix proteins, autogenous bone from an implant osteotomy site was placed in the defect. Complete fill of the defect with a hard bonelike substance was seen 3 months later when the adjacent implant was uncovered.

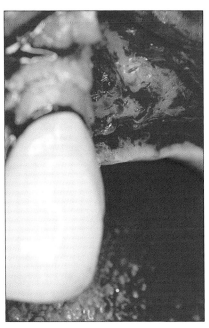

Fig 6-6a A deep one-wall defect was found on the distal aspect of the maxillary left canine.

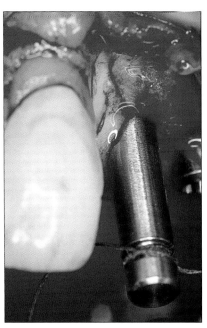

Fig 6-6b An osteotomy was performed for an implant, autogenous bone was harvested, and a directional marker was placed. Ethylenediaminetetraacetic acid is seen on the distal aspect of the tooth.

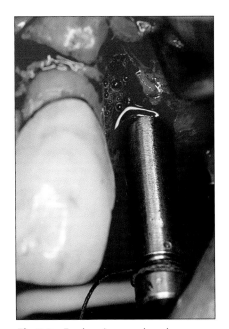

Fig 6-6c Emdogain was placed.

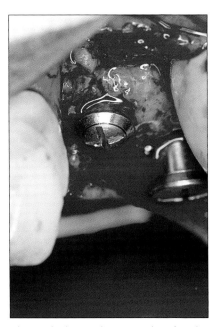

Fig 6-6d The implant was placed and a graft of autogenous bone used to maintain the flap position.

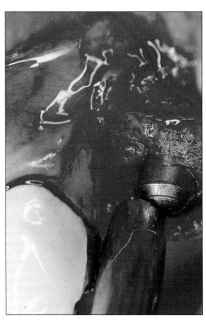

Fig 6-6e The flap was reopened 3 months later. A hard bonelike substance was found on the distal aspect of the canine.

Case 7 (Figs 6-7a to 6-7e)

Since enamel matrix proteins have shown the capacity to generate new attachment on denuded root surfaces, they can be applied to areas of gingival recession, as in this case.

The chief complaint of this 34-year-old woman was pain and tenderness in the mandibular anterior region. The recession on the right mandibular lateral incisor had substantially worsened recently. A full-thickness mucoperiosteal flap was raised and the tooth roots were planed and then treated with EDTA and enamel matrix proteins. The flap was coronally placed for a few minutes to allow the proteins to precipitate. A subepithelial connective graft was taken from the palate and covered with the flap.

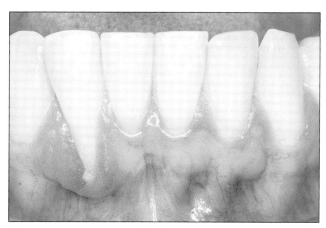

Fig 6-7a Patient presented with recession around the lateral incisor, which had progressed for some time.

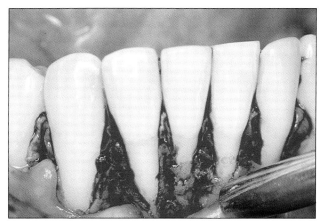

Fig 6-7b The area following flap elevation and planing of the lateral incisor root with profile reduction of the tooth.

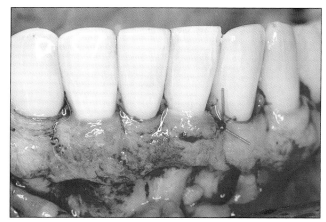

Fig 6-7c Emdogain and EDTA were placed and the flap re-placed to allow the Emdogain to precipitate on the root surface. A subepithelial connective tissue graft was then sutured into position and the previously elevated mucosal flap sutured over it.

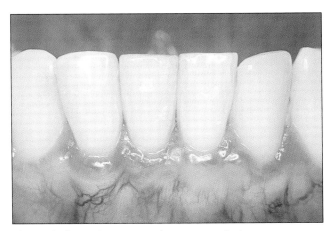

Fig 6-7d The graft area 3 weeks postoperatively.

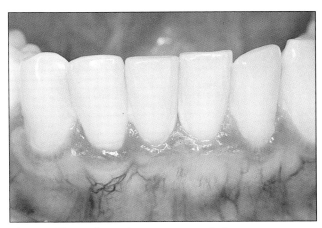

Fig 6-7e The graft area 1 year postoperatively.

Case 8 (Figs 6-8a and 6-8b)

This 30-year-old man complained of thermal sensitivity associated with gingival recession. Following several unsuccessful attempts to desensitize the area, surgery with subepithelial grafts and enamel matrix proteins was performed. (In the author's experience, soft tissue healing has often been enhanced by these proteins.) Any bone laid down in the area would be additionally beneficial. The healing proceeded uneventfully.

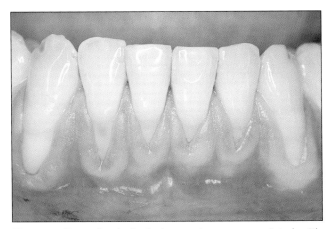

Fig 6-8a Generalized gingival recession was associated with thermal sensitivity. Emdogain was used as in Fig 6-7c.

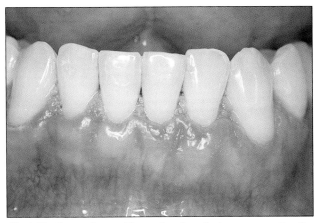

Fig 6-8b The graft area 18 months after placing a connective tissue graft and Emdogain.

Case 9 (Figs 6-9a to 6-9k)

Combining enamel matrix proteins with minimally invasive surgical techniques can have the advantage of enhanced healing with less trauma to the patient.

In this case, a 45-year-old woman had a deep pocket in the maxillary central incisor area, which caused esthetic concerns regarding treatment. In an attempt to reduce the probing depth to a minimum, the use of enamel matrix proteins was combined with surgery to produce a successful outcome.

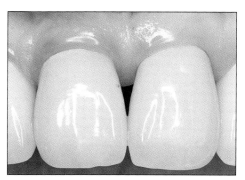

Fig 6-9a A patient with a two-wall bony defect in an area of esthetic concern.

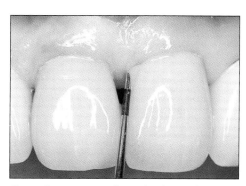

Fig 6-9b A 7-mm probing depth was found.

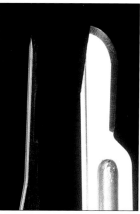

Fig 6-9c Microsurgical techniques, including instruments of reduced dimension, were used. A special scalpel blade compared with a #15 blade.

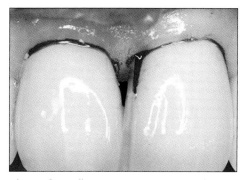

Fig 6-9d Smaller instruments were used along with minimal flap reflection to limit postoperative tissue shrinkage.

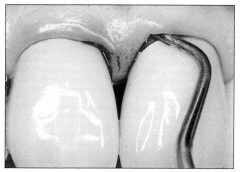

Fig 6-9e Sharp curettes were used for root planing.

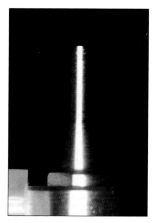

Fig 6-9f Specially designed instruments were used to remove granulation tissue.

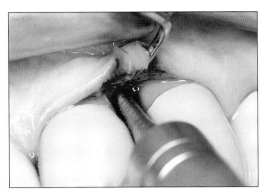

Fig 6-9g The degranulating device is pushed along the floor of the bony defect. (From Harrel SK. A minimally invasive surgical approach for periodontal bone grafting. Int J Periodont Restorative Dent 1998;18:161.)

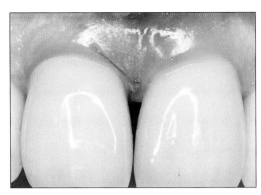

Fig 6-9h Following the use of EDTA and the placement of Emdogain, a single interproximal suture was used.

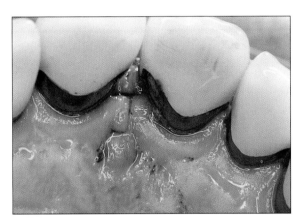

Fig 6-9i Palatal view of the suture.

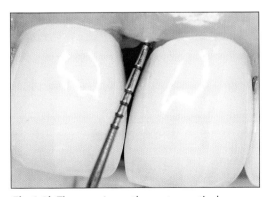

Fig 6-9j The area 4 months postoperatively.

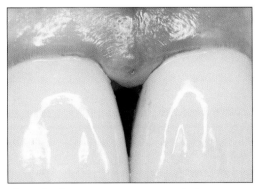

Fig 6-9k The area 1 year postoperatively.

Supportive Periodontal Treatment

Supportive periodontal treatment (SPT) is the preferred term for the continuation of periodontal therapy, previously termed "maintenance." It is performed by a dentist, although components of SPT can be performed by a dental hygienist under the supervision of the dentist.

Supportive periodontal treatment includes an update of medical and dental histories, radiographic review, extraoral and intraoral soft tissue examination, dental examination, periodontal evaluation, removal of bacterial plaque from the supragingival and subgingival regions, scaling and root planing where indicated, polishing of the teeth, and a review of the patient's plaque control efficacy.[1] These procedures are performed at selected intervals to assist the periodontal patient in maintaining oral health.

Supportive periodontal therapy follows active therapy, and the patient may move back into active care if the disease undergoes a period of exacerbation. The supportive phase begins after completion of active periodontal therapy and continues at varying intervals for the life of the dentition.

Recurrence of periodontal diseases can be prevented or limited by optimal personal oral hygiene[2,3] and/or periodic maintenance care.[4] Because patients rarely are completely effective in removing plaque accumulations,[5,6] SPT can reduce the chance of future attachment loss. Patients who have had regenerative procedures usually require frequent SPT because personal supragingival oral hygiene alone has not been shown to control attachment loss in these patients.[7–9]

The following sections describe a typical SPT visit.

Examination and Diagnosis

The visit begins with a chart review and an update of medical and dental histories. The dentist then performs a clinical examination and records the findings for comparison to previous baseline measurements. The elements of this examination are:

- Extraoral examination
- Dental examination including tooth mobility and fremitus; restorative, prosthetic, and dental caries assessments; tooth contacts, uneven marginal ridges, drifting, and so on
- Periodontal examination including probing depths (six per tooth)

Periapical and bite-wing radiographs are taken with a paralleling technique.[10] The clinical status of the disease determines the frequency and number of radiographs. A series of vertical bite-wing radiographs[11] or selected periapical or bite-wing radiographs can be used between full-mouth series.

Assessment of disease status is accomplished by comparing the clinical and radiographic findings with previous measurements. These may include:

- Comparison of probing depths *plus* gingival recession to reveal changes in probing depth and attachment level
- Assessment of bleeding on probing (the absence of bleeding usually indicates gingival health)

Finally, the dentist assesses the patient's personal oral hygiene status.

Therapy

The therapeutic phase of the visit consists of treatment, behavior modification, and evaluation of systemic risk factors. The dentist first removes subgingival plaque and calculus as well as supragingival deposits. He or she then provides education in behavior modification as necessary. Such education may include proper oral hygiene techniques; compliance with suggested SPT intervals; and counseling regarding other contributing factors, such as smoking cessation. Adjunctive antimicrobial agents may be administered or prescribed in a few select cases.[12]

Finally, the dentist evaluates the effect of any systemic risk factors on the patient's treatment plan. As needed, the dentist may encourage smoking cessation, discuss the patient's diabetic status, and establish the patient's Interleukin-1 genotype (if this was not done previously).

Communication

Two-way communication is important to the success of SPT. The dentist needs to keep patients apprised of their current status and explain any needed alterations in treatment. Open communication is also important between the dentist and the surgeon who will be performing additional care or participating in SPT.

Planning Treatment Schedules

Clinical Parameters

The scheduling of future treatment should be based on an evaluation of clinical findings and an assessment of disease status. These factors may alter the frequency of SPT or return the patient to active treatment.

Currently, the decision to return the patient to active therapy is based on increases in probing depth and bleeding on probing compared to a baseline.[13–15] This baseline is first established at the initial examination and again following active therapy. Unfortunately, increases in probing depth represent a measure of attachment loss that may no longer be active, and bleeding on probing indicates progressive disease only in a small percentage of cases.

In general, those individuals who have poor oral hygiene and systemic risk factors should receive SPT more frequently. As more is learned about diagnosing disease activity, this information should be used to help set SPT intervals and make decisions on returning the patient to active therapy.

Frequency of Intervals

Numerous studies have shown that less attachment loss occurs and fewer teeth are lost when patients maintain regular SPT intervals[3,4,16–32] as compared to patients who are seen less often[33–35] or not at all.[36–39] Occasionally, despite the best efforts of clinicians and patients, some individuals may lose teeth despite maintaining a regular SPT schedule.[40–42] This group of individuals may benefit from additional diagnostic procedures such as microbial analysis and therapy that includes antimicrobial agents.[43,44]

For patients with a previous history of periodontitis, results from a number of clinical trials suggest that the frequency of SPT should be less than 6 months. Intervals of 2 weeks,[23,45] 2 to 3 months,[16] 3 months,[4,17,34,46–51] 3 to 4 months,[3,21] 3 to 6 months,[13,18,52] and 4 to 6 months[40] have been proposed and studied. These data indicate that SPT intervals of at least four times a year will result in a decreased likelihood of progressive disease as compared to patients seen less frequently.[13,16,19,25,26] Those individuals who have undergone procedures for regeneration generally show a propensity for periodontitis and therefore usually need more frequent SPT.

Compliance with suggested SPT intervals can affect the success of treatment. Patients treated for periodontitis who comply with suggested SPT intervals will experience less attachment loss and tooth loss than patients who do not comply with the schedule.[24,34,39,53–55]

The time required for SPT appointments should be dictated by the number of teeth present, the local environment (eg, access, the type and history of disease, distribution and depth of the sulci), patient cooperation, and frequency of SPT visits.[16] Typically, a visit for a patient with a history of periodontitis will require one hour. Patients with advanced attachment loss associated with periodontitis or rapidly progressive forms of periodontitis generally should be seen in the periodontist's office for SPT, with the general dentist maintaining the nonperiodontal aspects of the dentition.

Summary

Supportive periodontal treatment is an essential part of the treatment of inflammatory periodontal diseases. It provides removal of the microbial challenge and is essential to long-term stabilization of patients who have received regenerative treatment for these diseases. For patients with a past history of periodontitis, four or more visits per year are usually required. Until risk detection for future attachment loss becomes more precise, these patients should be seen on a routine basis for evaluation of clinical parameters. The SPT interval should be established with consideration of research findings and individual clinical measures.

References

1. American Academy of Periodontology. Current Terminology for Periodontics and Insurance Reporting Manual, ed 6. Chicago: American Academy of Periodontology, 1991:22.

2. Löe H, Theilade E, Jensen SB. Experimental gingivitis in man. J Periodontol 1965;36:177.

3. Suomi JD, Greene JC, Vermillion JR, Doyle J, Chang J, Leatherwood EC. The effect of controlled oral hygiene procedures on the progression of periodontal disease in adults: Results after third and final year. J Periodontol 1971;42:152.

4. Ramfjord SP, Morrison EC, Burgett FG, et al. Oral hygiene and maintenance of periodontal support. J Periodontol 1982;53(1):26.

5. Johansson LA, Oster B, Hamp SE. Evaluation of cause-related periodontal therapy and compliance with maintenance care recommendations. J Clin Periodontol 1984;11(10):689.

6. Wilson TG. Compliance. A review of the literature with possible applications to periodontics. J Periodontol 1987;58(10):706.

7. Weigel C, Bragger U, Hammerle CHF, Mombelli A, Lang NP. Maintenance of new attachment 1 and 4 years following guided tissue regeneration (GTR). J Clin Periodontol 1995;22(9):661.

8. Gottlow J, Nyman S, Karring T. Maintenance of new attachment gained through guided tissue regeneration. J Clin Periodontol 1992;19:315.

9. Cortellini P, Pini-Prato G, Tonetti M. Periodontal regeneration of human infrabony defect (V). Effect of oral hygiene on long-term stability. J Clin Periodontol 1994;21:606.

10. Ramfjord SP. Design of studies or clinical trials to evaluate the effectiveness of agents or procedures for the prevention or treatment of loss of the periodontium. J Periodontal Res 1974;9(suppl):78.

11. Updegrave WJ. Vertical interproximal radiography. Dent Radiogr Photogr 1978;51:56.

12. Ciancio SC. Chemotherapeutic agents and periodontal therapy—their impact on clinical practice. J Periodontol 1986;57:18.

13. Haffajee AD, Socransky SS, Smith C, Dibart S. Relation of baseline microbial parameters to future periodontal attachment loss. J Clin Periodontol 1991;18:744.

14. Chace R. Retreatment in periodontal practice. J Periodontol 1977;48(7):410.

15. Mombelli A. Treatment of recurrent periodontal disease by root planing and Ornidazole (Tiberal). Clinical and microbiological findings. J Clin Periodontol 1989;16(1):38.

16. Axelsson P, Lindhe J. The significance of maintenance care in the treatment of periodontal disease. J Clin Periodontol 1981;8(4):281.

17. Knowles J, Burgett F, Nissle R, Shick R, Morrison E, Ramfjord S. Results of periodontal treatment related to pocket depth and attachment level. Eight years. J Periodontol 1979;50(5):225.

18. Lindhe J, Nyman S. Long-term maintenance of patients treated for advanced periodontal disease. J Clin Periodontol 1984;11(8):504.

19. Ramfjord S, Caffesse R, Morrison E, et al. Four modalities of periodontal treatment compared over five years. J Periodontal Res 1987;22(3):222.

20. Westfeld E, Nyman S, Socransky S, Lindhe J. Significance of frequency of professional tooth cleaning for healing following periodontal surgery. J Clin Periodontol 1983;10:148.

21. Pihlström BL, McHugh RB, Oliphant TH, Ortiz-Campos C. Comparison of surgical and nonsurgical treatment of periodontal disease. A review of current studies and additional results after 6 1/2 years. J Clin Periodontol 1983;10(5):524.

22. Badersten A, Nilvéus R, Egelberg J. Effects of nonsurgical periodontal therapy. II. Severely advanced periodontitis. J Clin Periodontol 1984;11(1):63.

23. Nyman S, Rosling B, Lindhe J. Effect of professional tooth cleaning on healing after periodontal surgery. J Clin Periodontol 1975;2(2):80.

24. Becker W, Berg L, Becker BE. The long-term evaluation of periodontal maintenance in 95 patients. Int J Periodontics Restorative Dent 1984;2:55.

25. Axelsson P, Lindhe J. Effect of controlled oral hygiene procedures on caries and periodontal disease in adults. J Clin Periodontol 1978;5(2):133.

26. Axelsson P, Lindhe J. Effect of controlled oral hygiene procedures on caries and periodontal disease in adults: Results after 6 years. J Clin Periodontol 1981;8(3):239.

27. Brandzaeg P, Jamison HC. The effect of controlled cleansing of teeth on periodontal health and oral hygiene in Norwegian Army recruits. J Periodontol 1964;35:302.

28. Chawla TN, Nanda RS, Kapoor KK. Dental prophylaxis procedures in control of periodontal disease in Lucknow (rural) India. J Periodontol 1975;46:498.

29. Lövdal A, Arno A, Schei O, Waerhaug J. Combined effect of subgingival scaling and controlled oral hygiene on the incidence of gingivitis. Acta Odontol Scand 1961;19:537.

30. Schallhorn RG, Snider LE. Periodontal maintenance therapy. J Am Dent Assoc 1981;103(2):227.

31. Jendresen MD, Hamilton MA, McLean JW, Phillips RW, Ramfjord SP. Report of the committee on scientific investigation of the American Academy of Restorative Dentistry. J Prosthet Dent 1984;51:823.

32. Kaldahl WB, Kalkwarf KL, Patil KD, Dyer JK, Bates RE. Evaluation of four modalities of periodontal therapy. Mean probing depth, probing attachment level and recession changes. J Periodontol 1988;59(12):783.

33. American Academy of Periodontology. In: World Workshop in Clinical Periodontics. Chicago: American Academy of Periodontology, 1989:IX–24.

34. Wilson TG, Glover ME, Malik AK, Schoen JA, Dorsett D. Tooth loss in maintenance patients in a private periodontal practice. J Periodontol 1987;58(4):231.

35. DeVore CH, Duckworth DM, Beck FM, Hicks MJ, Brumfield FW, Horton JE. Bone loss following periodontal therapy in subjects without frequent periodontal maintenance. J Periodontol 1986;57:354.

36. Nyman S, Lindhe J, Rosling B. Periodontal surgery in plaque-infected dentitions. J Clin Periodontol 1977;4(4):240.

37. Becker W, Berg L, Becker BE. Untreated periodontal disease: A longitudinal study. J Periodontol 1979;50(5):234.

38. Lindhe J, Haffajee AD, Socransky SS. Progression of periodontal disease in adult subjects in the absence of periodontal therapy. J Clin Periodontol 1983;10(4):433.

39. Becker W, Becker BE, Berg LE. Periodontal treatment without maintenance. A retrospective study in 44 patients. J Periodontol 1984;55(9):505.

40. Hirschfeld L, Wasserman B. A long-term survey of tooth loss in 600 treated periodontal patients. J Periodontol 1978;49(5):225.

41. McFall WT Jr. Tooth loss in 100 treated patients with periodontal disease. A long-term study. J Periodontal 1982;53(9):539.

42. Meador H, Love J, Suddick P. The long-term effectiveness of periodontal therapy in a clinical practice. J Periodontol 1985;56:253.

43. Douglass CW, Fox CH. Determining the value of a periodontal diagnostic test. J Periodontol 1991;62:721.

44. van Winkelhoff A, Tijhof C, de Graf J. Microbiological and clinical results of metronidazole plus amoxicillin therapy in Actinobacillus actinomycetemcomitans-associated periodontitis. J Periodontol 1992;63:52.

45. Rosling B, Nyman S, Lindhe J, Jern B. The healing potential of the periodontal tissues following different techniques of periodontal surgery in plaque-free dentitions. A 2-year clinical study. J Clin Periodontol 1976;3(4):233.

46. Ramfjord SP, Knowles JW, Nissle RR, Burgett FG, Shick RA. Results following three modalities of periodontal therapy. J Periodontol 1975;46(9):522.

47. Fleszar TJ, Knowles JW, Morrison EC, Burgett FG, Nissle RR, Ramfjord SP. Tooth mobility and periodontal therapy. J Clin Periodontol 1980;7(6):495.

48. Hill RW, Ramfjord SP, Morrison EC, et al. Four types of periodontal treatment over two years. J Periodontol 1981;52:655.

49. Becker W, Becker BE, Ochsenbein C, et al. A longitudinal study comparing scaling, osseous surgery and modified Widman procedures—Results after one year. J Periodontol 1988;59(6):351.

50. Ramfjord SP, Knowles JW, Nissle RR, Shick RA, Burgett FG. Longitudinal study of periodontal therapy. J Periodontol 1973;44:66.

51. Oliver RC. Tooth loss with and without periodontal therapy. Periodontal Abstr 1969;17:8.

52. Lindhe J, Nyman S. The effect of plaque control and surgical pocket elimination on the establishment and maintenance of periodontal health. A longitudinal study of periodontal therapy in cases of advanced disease. J Clin Periodontol 1975;2(2):67.

53. Kerr NW. Treatment of chronic periodontitis. 45% failure rate after 5 years. Brit Dent J 1981;150(8):222.

54. Duckworth J, Brose M, Avers R, French C, Savitt E. Therapeutic implications of the bacterial pathogens associated around dental implants. J Dent Res 1987;66:114.

55. Mendoza A, Newcomb G, Nixon K. Compliance with supportive periodontal therapy. J Periodontol 1991;62:731.